HACKING YOUR HEALTH
3 WEEK DETOX

PRESENTED BY:

*Thrive*CLEAN

WHY I CREATED THIS JOURNAL FOR YOU

Hi there! I am Tiffany Hinton, the GF Mom Certified. As a functional medicine practicioner, I have met many women over the last several years who struggle with trying to figur eout what to eat and how to make a transition to clean eating.

As an autoimmune disease survivor and after years of struggling to figure out I had Celiac, Endometriosis, Crohns and food allergies, I found the magic in the kitchen. Our family started to thrive. We found our healing through the power of food, and you can too!

My story is long and the struggle for better health was real. I remember my symptoms began at the age of fourteen. I was the child with acid reflux, bloat and stomach complaints. By the time I was eighteen my intestines were bleeding. I was diagnosed with IBS and Ulcerative Colitis. My condition and symptoms continued to get worse. At one point in my mid-twenties I was taking 25 pills a day, struggled to stay awake during the day and was in constant pain. Imagine a charlie horse in your gut. Except this one you cannot rub out or stretch away.

When I was in my late twenties I was rushed to the ER and had an emergency appendectomy. The ER surgeon informed me he had removed my appendix, not because it had ruptured, bu because it was being choked by an unknown tissue. My body was trying to kill my appendix. My firs thought was cancer. grammar fi paragraph 1: By the way, this is how my husband got to meet m

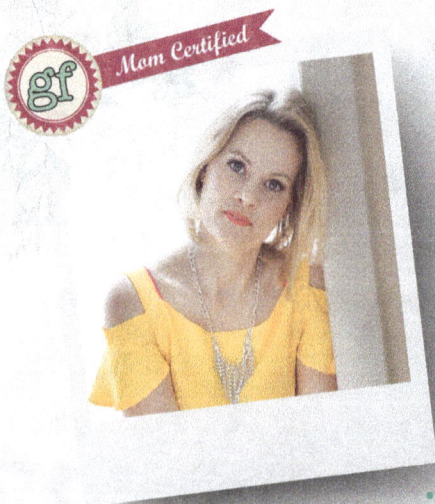

Mom Certified
gf

arents for the first time; in the R at 3:30 a.m. Welcome to the amily, right!?

earned my appendix was being ompressed by endrometrial ssue, and I was diagnosed ith stage 4 endrometriosis. ly health continued to decline nd I was also suffering from nexplained infertility which I truggled with for over 14 years.

remember the day I came ome from the OB in tears and ny husband said, "call his boss." O BACK! We did just that and learned they did not

have a specialty in my case and would no longer be able to treat or see me as a patient. At this point we were over a half million dollars in debt from my medical expenses. So, where do you turn? GOOGLE of course!

I found a board certified doctor in both my disease and Endocrinology. I remember my first visit clearly. I showed up with a binder and was there to interview him for the job of healing me. He had me tested for 200 different diseases. This came as a surprise and frustration. Dr. Rana explained he could not treat me if we did not know the cause. To my surprise I was positive for the celiac antibodies. I went home from that appointment with a list of foods I could eat. This was my saving grace. I was not to consume gluten, dairy or sugar for at least 1 year to allow my body time to heal. We ate a lot of veggies and chicken. What I didn't know at the time, but now realize, was that Dr. Rana was treating me with functional medicine. Within 9 months I was pregnant with our first daughter, Franki. God blessed us with 3 kids in less than 3 years.

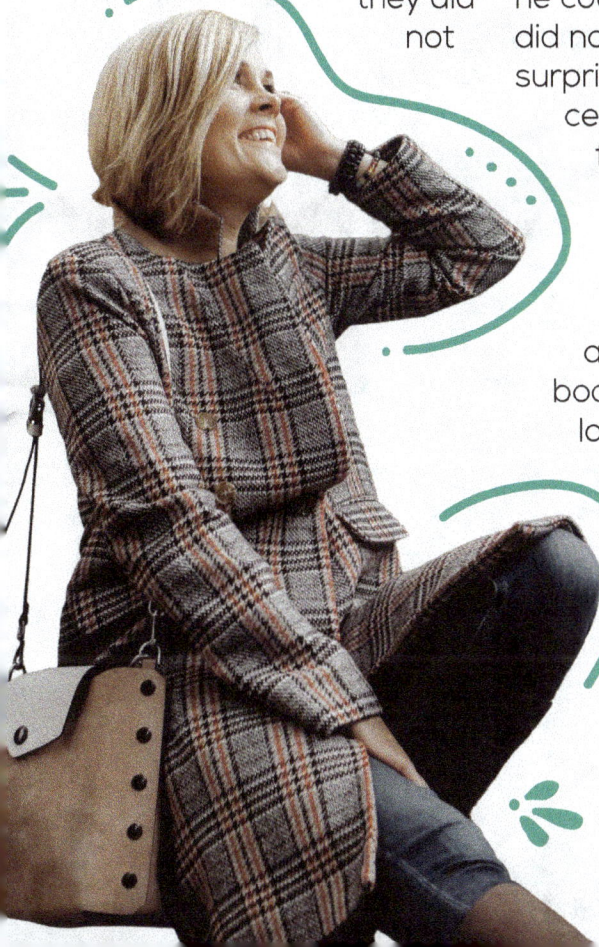

All of our children have food allergies and Lillie is also diagnosed with Celiac and Crohns Disease like myself.

In December 2013 when I was pregnant with Josi, my uterus and colon fused and became one organ. When I went into labor with her they both ruptured. I was rushed into emergency surgery and while still awake they began to cauterize both organs and put me back together. God saved my life that day because he had bigger plans for me.

In October of 2014, I was back at the gastroenterologist office because my colon was acting up and not functioning. The colonoscopy showed that it had died in places where it had been cauterized. I had my second colon resection surgery. I never filled the scripts because I knew the power of food. I went home that day with prescriptions written and called our local functional medicine doctor who helped me heal. This is what lead me to move from just writing cookbooks and designing recipes to helping other women have a life and a body they love.

Together we can succeed. I want to help you, and all you have to do is raise your hand and say, "Me too! I want to be more. I want to love life and my body."

I encourage you to take this journey with me into a life of clean eating and a thriving lifestyle filled with restoring your health.

FOLLOW TIFFANY HINTON

HEALING STARTS HERE

➤ HERE ➤

ARE YOU READY?

TABLE OF CONTENTS

MINDSET

WEEK 1

WEEK 2

WEEK 3

ADRENAL RESET WEEK

THE BEST WAY
TO GET SOMETHING
DONE IS TO
BEGIN

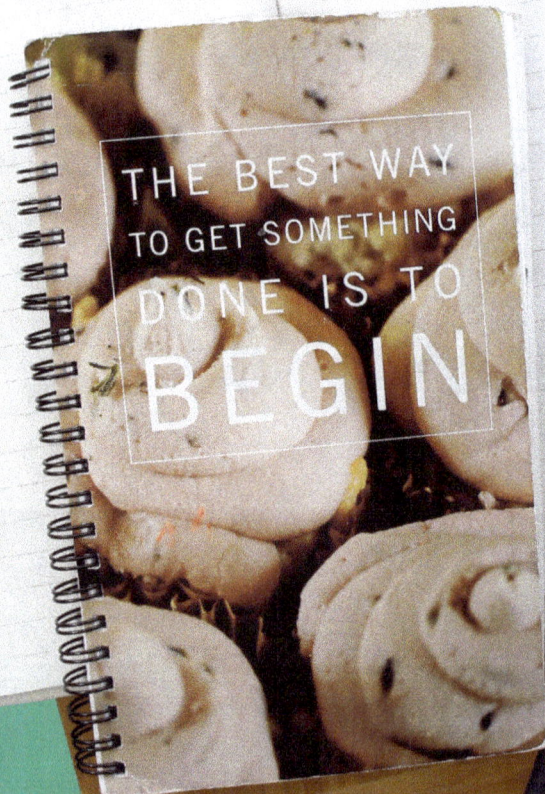

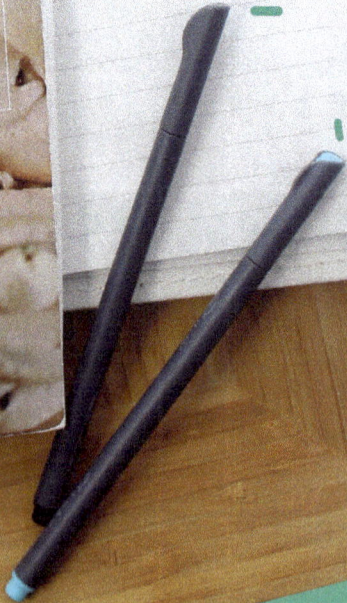

MINDSET

✣ TIPS FOR A ✣ SUCCESSFUL WEEK

- Always read labels. Don't assume food is "clean". For example, some nut butters contain added oils. Look for nut butters with nuts only without the added oils. Read labels on all foods that have a label...only exceptions are whole foods (fruit, vegetables, fresh meats, etc). Hidden ingredients can include sugar, soy, high fructose, corn syrup, starch, etc.

- Select green or non-starchy vegetables such as broccoli, spinach, green beans, squash, carrots, brussel sprouts, etc. Corn, peas, and lima beans are not an option in this week's choices.

- Buy organic fruit, vegetables and meats if/when possible and your budget allows.

- If you don't like a meal for that day, simply substitute it for another meal/snack you like on the plan

- NO SODA - keep ALCOHOL to a minimum if you HAVE to drink it at all.

- 1 Cup of Black Coffee is allowed each day.

- Aim to drink at least half of your body weight in ounces OR 1 gallon of water a day!(Adding lemon acts as a diuretic to rid excess water weight and helps eliminate heartburn)

- No extra snacks/treats. Follow this to a "T" and you'll feel better in 5 days!

5 STEPS TO SUCCESS

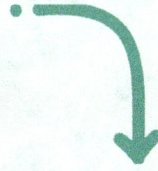

1

FOOD
- 4 oz protein
- 1 to 2 cups fruit including berries
- Bone broth to help heal the gut

2

WATER
- Goal this week is 75 oz a day. Try carrying a water bottle with you.

3

EXERCISE
- 20 minutes a day for cell regeneration

4

DECLUTTER
- Throw, give, or donate 1 item everyday

5

EPSOM SALT SOAK
- 20 minutes 3 times a week

MINDSET MUST-HAVES

AUDIBLE

Audible is the leading creator and provider of premium audio storytelling, enriching the lives of our millions of listeners every day. With our customer-centric approach to technological innovation and superior programming, Audible has reinvented a media category, and is the driving force behind today's audio entertainment revolution.

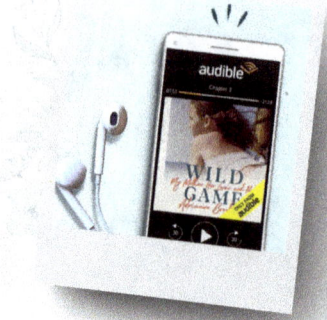

TINYURL.COM/GFMOMAUDIBLE

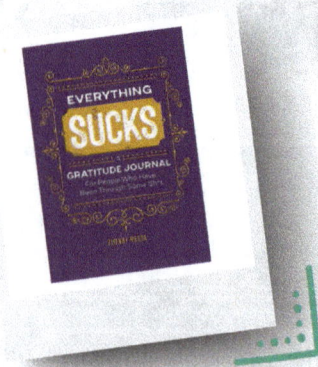

EVERYTHING SUCKS: A GRAT-ITUDE JOURNAL FOR PEOPLE WHO HAVE BEEN THROUGH SOME SH*T

You don't always have to be grateful. Some days (or months, or decades) you just aren't feeling it. But feeling it a little more often couldn't hurt, right? Everything Sucks is your judgement-free space for dragging yourself down the path of positivity and gratitude kicking and screaming if need be.

TINYURL.COM/GFMOMEVERYTHINGSUCKS

WHAT ARE YOUR MUST-HAVES?

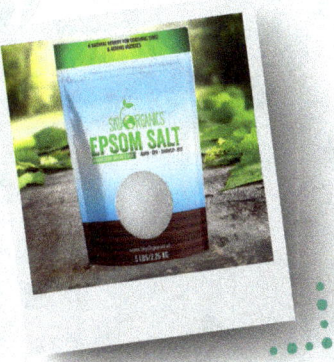

SKY ORGANIC'S EPSOM SALT

Use Sky Organics Epsom Salt as a comforting bath soak to comfort muscles after workouts, remove impurities, and unwind in the tub. Our Epsom Salt is GMO-free, Kosher, USP grade, vegan, and cruelty-free.

tinyurl.com/gfmomepsomsalt

PALEOVALLEY: NEUROEFFECT

Help fuel your brain for supported concentration, clarity, and brain function. The ingredients in NeuroEffect have shown to support levels of BDNF, a key neuro-protein which works as a fertilizer for the brain. This gives you a safe, organic supplement alternative that can help you with work, studying, or other daily tasks.

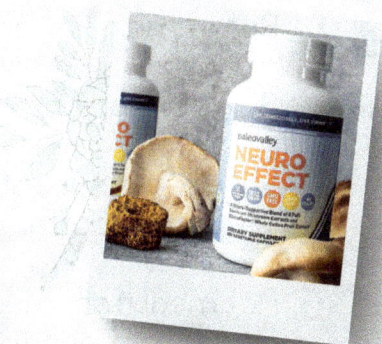

TINYURL.COM/GFMOMPALEO

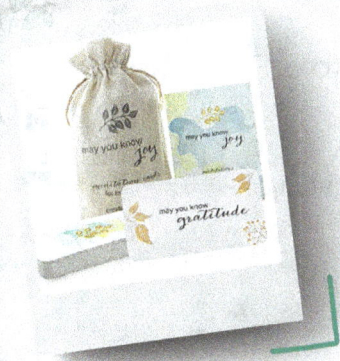

MAY YOU KNOW JOY

The Seeds of Intention card set is a beautiful way to inspire our best living. The card deck offers inspirational prompts, and the gift set includes a gorgeous bark card stand and rose quartz crystal for energy clearing and to promote self-love.

TINYURL.COM/GFMOMJOY

❧ THE DAILY PLAN ❧

- Smoothie

- Berries with flax or nuts/seeds

- Salad jar for lunch - full of flavor and veggies
-
- Veggie and nut butter or fruit with nut butter like peanut butter (sugar free)

- Hot meal from menu, these feed up to 4 people, no need to cook 2 meals at home

- Smoothie for dessert (optional)

- Overnight fast to allow the liver to detox and the cells to start to heal without impact

- No extra snacks/treats. Follow this to a "T" and you'll feel better in 5 days!

Fill in with raw nuts, including pecans, if you are still hungry

WEEK 1

DETOX FAQ

Q: I am allergic or do not like something on the meal plan. What do I do?

A: You can either substitute the item for something comparable (veggie for a veggie, peanut butter for other nut butter), eliminate the item (if possible), or substitute for another meal in the same category (breakfast for breakfast, lunch for lunch, dinner for dinner).

Q: Do I have to follow the meal plan exactly?

A: No, you do not have to eat the meals on the exact days they are planned. Everybody is busy and we want you to make this plan work for you. If Day 1 dinner is chicken, but you want the beef meal instead, you can do that. However, please try to choose only meals from the plan.

Q: I am a Vegetarian. What do I do?

A: Substitute an equal calorie item with the same amount of protein for any of the meat items on the menu. (Tempeh, Tofu, etc.)

Q: This is a lot of food. Do I have to eat all of it?

A: We recommend eating all 5 meals (3 meals and 2 snacks). However, listen to your body. If you are just too full to finish a meal, don't force it.

Q: I'm still hungry. Should I eat more?

A: In most cases, this should be enough food for each day. Make sure you are drinking enough water since dehydration can lead to a feeling of hunger. Men may need to add a little more protein or carbs per meal.

Q: Can I still juice?

A: It should be fine to keep juicing. Just remember, depending on the juicer, eating whole fruit is actually better for you. Sometimes juicing doesn't always include the important pulp/fiber. Also, juicing 5 apples for your meal really isn't that healthy. It is a lot of sugar, even if it is natural sugars.

Q: I'm going through withdrawals from soda. What should I do?

A: Drink a lot of water and hang in there. It will pass and you will feel so much better at the end of the week!

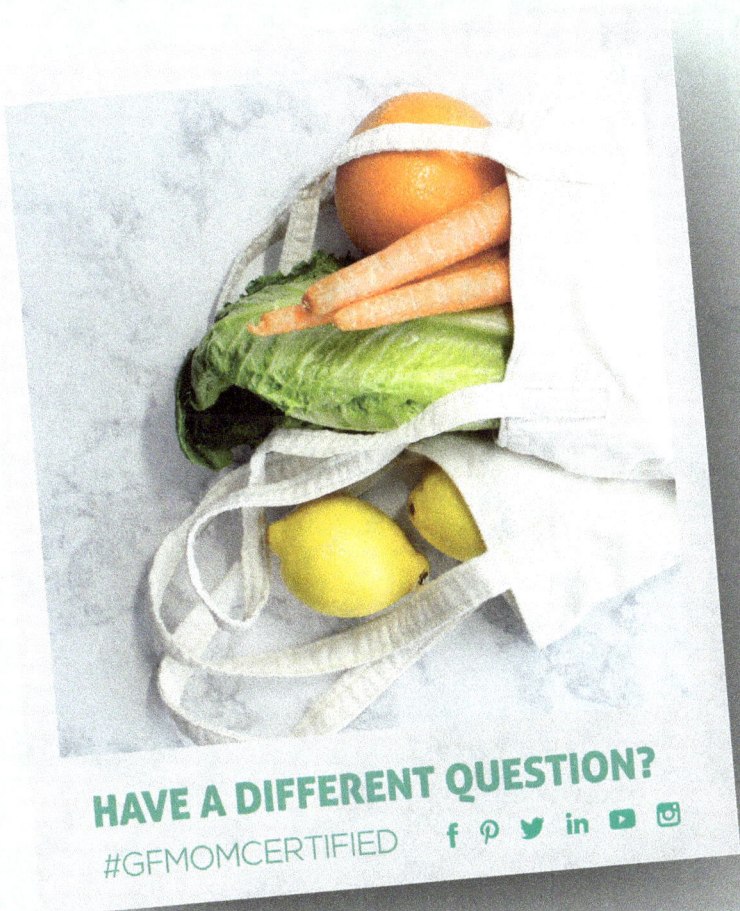

HAVE A DIFFERENT QUESTION?
#GFMOMCERTIFIED f P y in ▶ ⊙

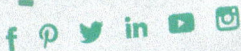

WEEK 1 MENU

	MON	TUE	WED	THU	FRI
BREAKFAST	Strawberry Banana Smoothie	Strawberry Banana Smoothie	Chocolate Banana Almond Smoothie	Strawberry Banana Smoothie	Chocolate Banana Almond Smoothie
AM SNACK	Berry Mix Salad	Berry Mix Salad	Banana Apple Muffin	Banana Apple Muffin	Green Apple and Almond Butter
LUNCH	Little Italy Salad in a Jar	Mixed Green Salad with Almonds	Simple Spinach Salad	Southwest Turbo Salad	Salad in a Jar
PM SNACK	Green Apple and Almond Butter	Carrots and Almond Butter	Carrots and Roasted Red Hummus	Carrots and Roasted Red Hummus	Green Peppers and Roasted Red Hummus
DINNER	Veggie Curry Over Sweet Potato	Veggie Stir-Fry	Baked Stuffed Sweet Potato	Roasted Chicken Bites and Veggies	Pizza and Salad

✓	GROCERY LIST	QTY
☐	Packages of Strawberries (Freeze 1)	2
☐	Packages of Raspberries (Freeze 1)	2
☐	Package of Blackberries	1
☐	Package of Blueberries	1
☐	Oranges	4
☐	Lemons	4
☐	Granny Smith Apples	4
☐	Bundle of Spotted Bananas	1
☐	Heads of Lettuce	2
☐	Mixed Greens	1
☐	Bunches of Spinach	2
☐	Celery Package	1
☐	Cucumbers	2
☐	Zucchinis	2
☐	Red Bell Peppers	5
☐	Green Bell Peppers	3
☐	Red Onions	5
☐	Sweet Potatoes	4
☐	Baby Carrots	1

✓	GROCERY LIST	QTY
☐	Snap Peas	1
☐	Fresh Green Beans	1
☐	Fresh Ginger	1
☐	Head of Broccoli	1
☐	Garlic Bulbs	2
☐	Tomatoes	9
☐	Cherry Tomatoes	1
☐	Avocados	3
☐	Fresh Cilantro	1
☐	Fresh Basil	1
☐	Portabella Mushrooms	5
☐	Gallons of Coconut Milk	2.5
☐	Eggs	3
☐	Ground Flax	1
☐	Almond Butter	1
☐	Chicken Breasts	2
☐	lb of Sliced Pepperoni	1
☐	Cans of Chickpeas	2
☐	Can of Black Beans	1

PANTRY STAPLES

Potato Starch

Coconut Flour

Cocoa Powder

Himalayan Salt

Chili Powder

Pepper

Cumin

Coriander

Oregano

Turmeric

Chole Masala

Red Pepper Flakes

Aqua Fava
(Bean Water)

Namaste Muffin Mix

CONDIMENTS

Olive Oil

Grapeseed Oil

Coconut Oil

Sesame Oil

Raw Honey

Apple Cider Vinegar

Balsamic Vinegar

Rice Vinegar

Maple Syrup

Pesto

Sriracha

Spicy Mustard
(Non-GMO/Sugar
Free)

Braggs Liquid
Aminos

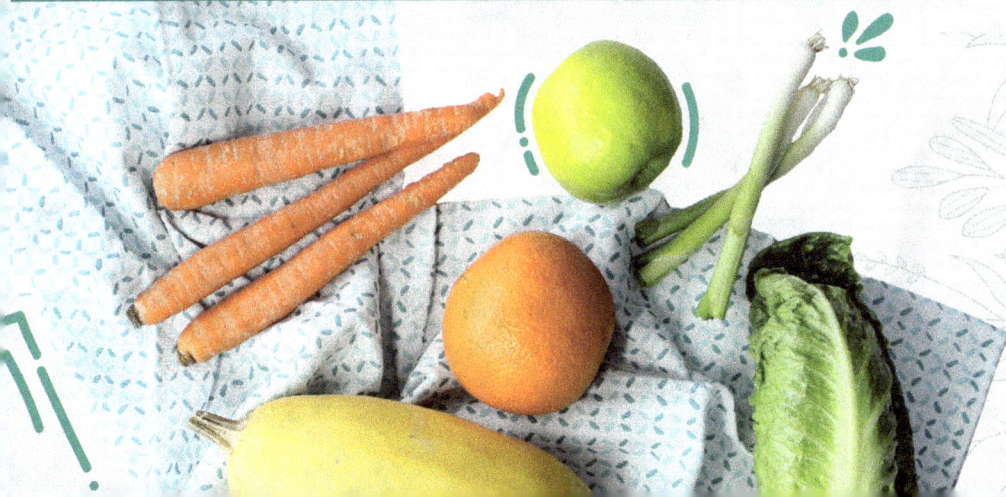

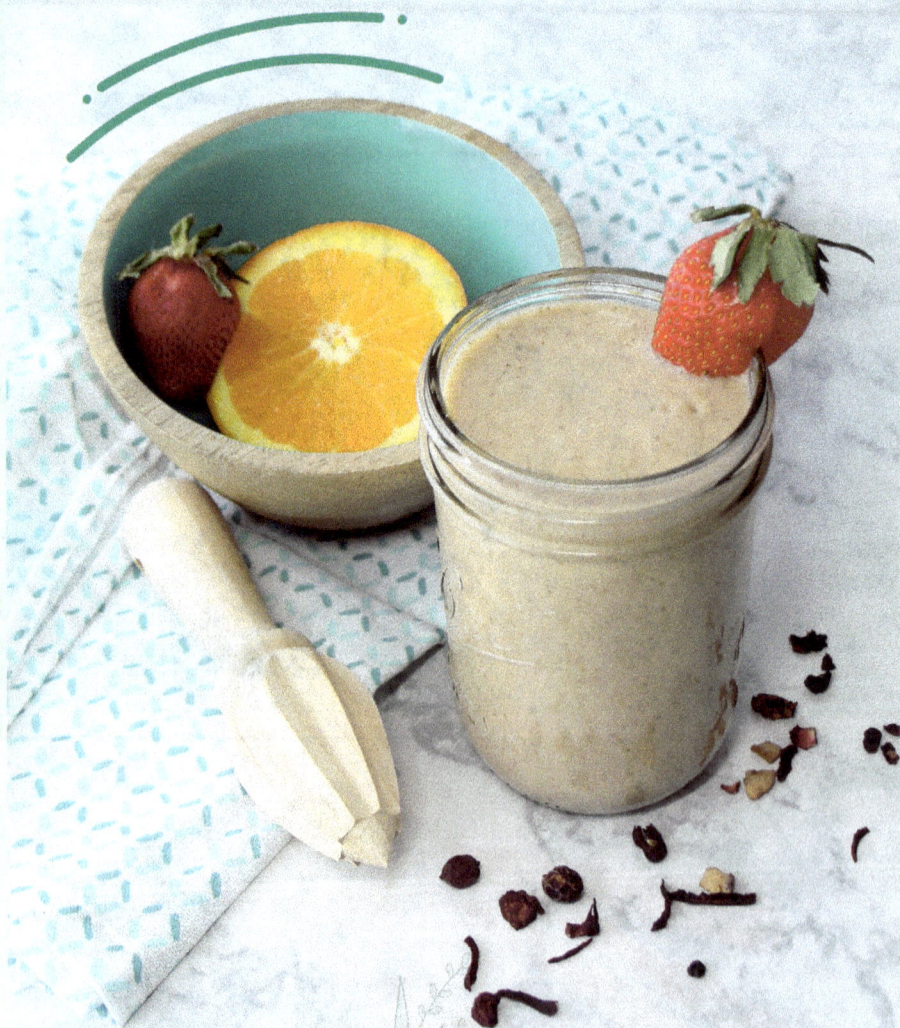

STRAWBERRY BANANA SMOOTHIE

INGREDIENTS

- 1/2 Cup Unsweetened Coconut Milk
- 1/2 Cup Frozen Strawberries
- 1/2 Orange
- 1 Brown Spotted Banana
- 1 Tsp Flax

DIRECTIONS

- Place all ingredients in blender and blend until creamy. The more ice or frozen berries, the thicker it gets.

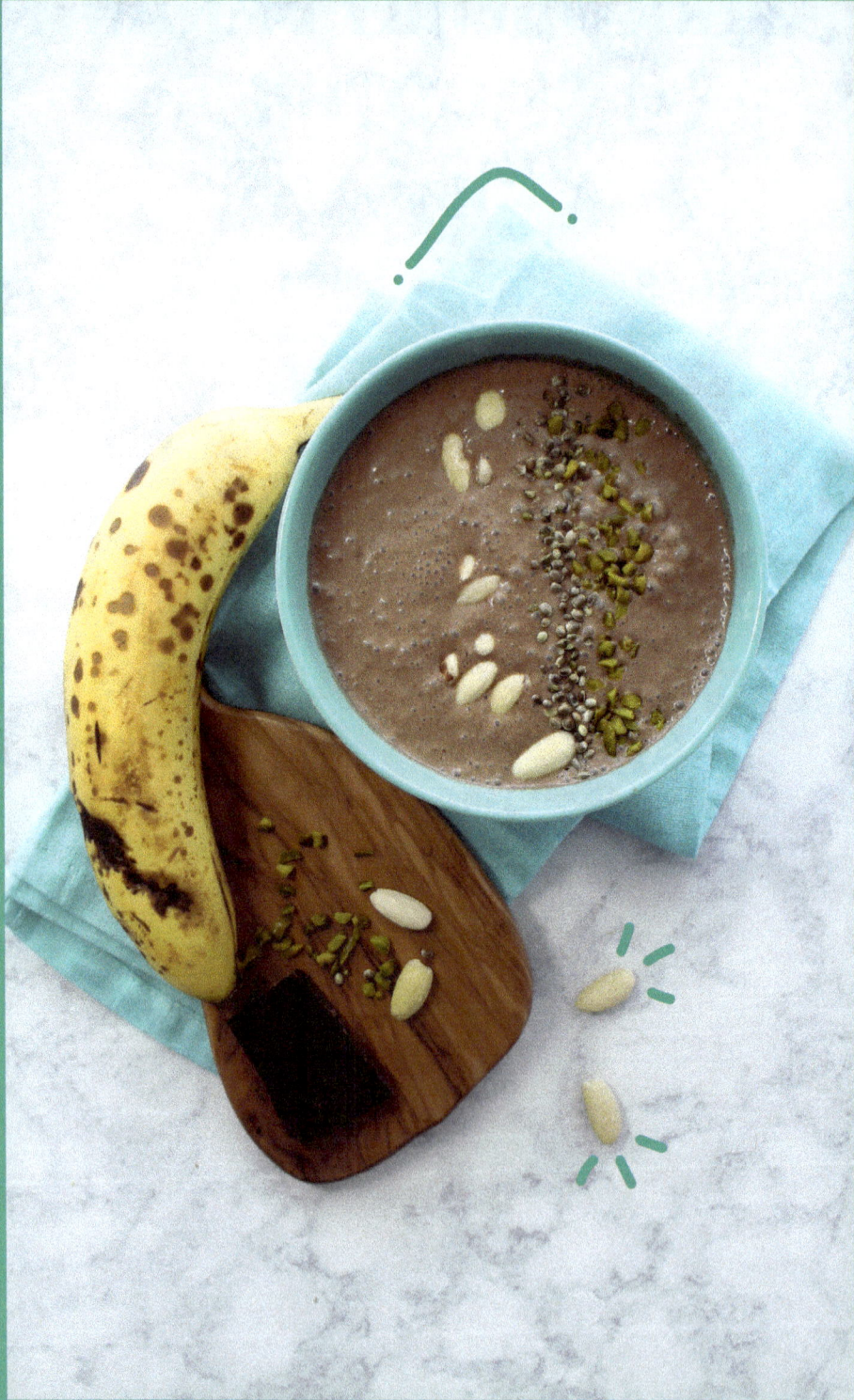

CHOCOLATE BANANA ALMOND SMOOTHIE

INGREDIENTS

- 1 Tbsp Cacao or Cocoa Powder
- 1 Tbsp Natural Almond Butter
- 1 Banana
- 1 Cup Coconut Milk
- 1/2 Cup Ice
- 1 Tsp Flax

DIRECTIONS

- Place all ingredients in blender and blend until creamy. The more ice or frozen berries, the thicker it gets.

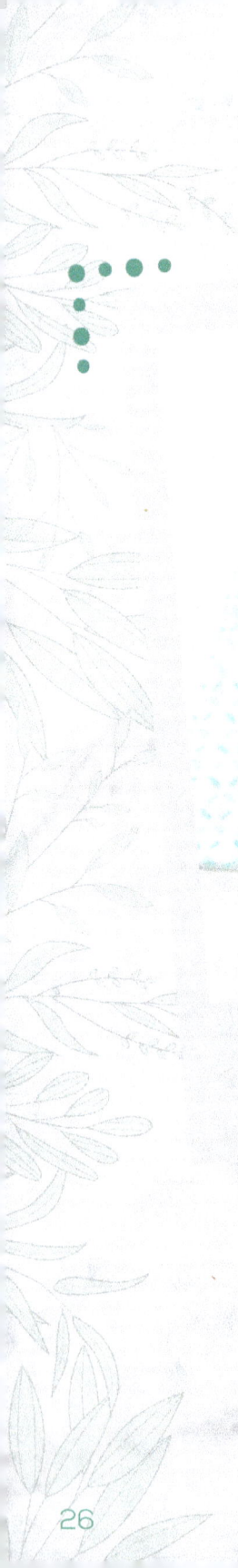

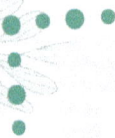

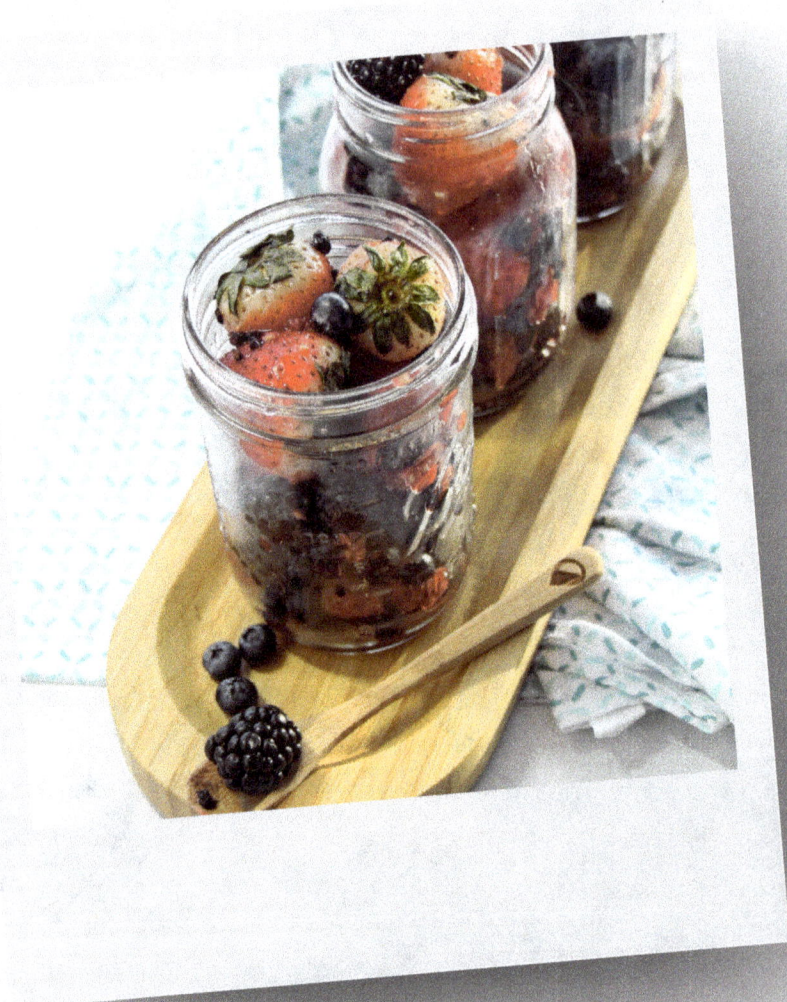

YUM! ←

BERRY MIX SALAD

INGREDIENTS

- 1 Package Strawberries, rinsed and halved
- 1 Package Raspberries, rinsed
- 1 Package Blackberries, rinsed
- 1 Package Blueberries, rinsed
- 2 Tbsp Ground Flax

DIRECTIONS

- Mix all the berries and fruit together in a large bowl and store covered in the fridge.

<u>Single Serving</u>
1 Cup Salad
1 Tsp Ground Flax

*tip alert: Try and dry off as much water as possible. This will help the fruit last longer in the fridge.

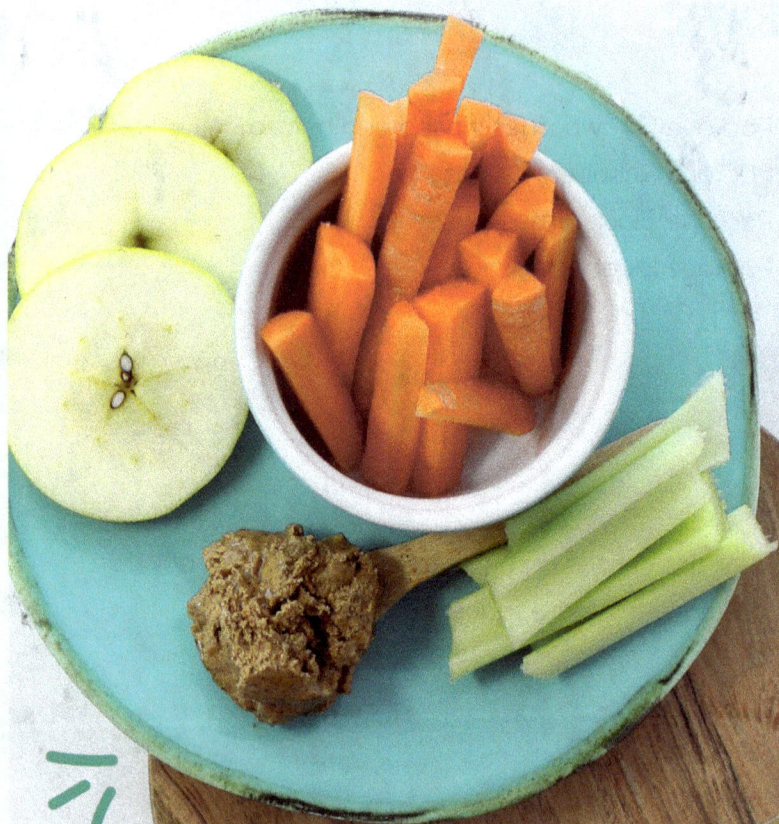

CARROTS AND ALMOND BUTTER

INGREDIENTS

- 10 Carrot Slices or Baby Carrrots
- 1 Tbsp Almond Butter

DIRECTIONS

- Dip carrots in almond butter and enjoy.

APPLE AND ALMOND BUTTER

INGREDIENTS

- 1 Green Apple, sliced
- 1 Tbsp Almond Butter

DIRECTIONS

- Dip apple slices in almond butter and enjoy.

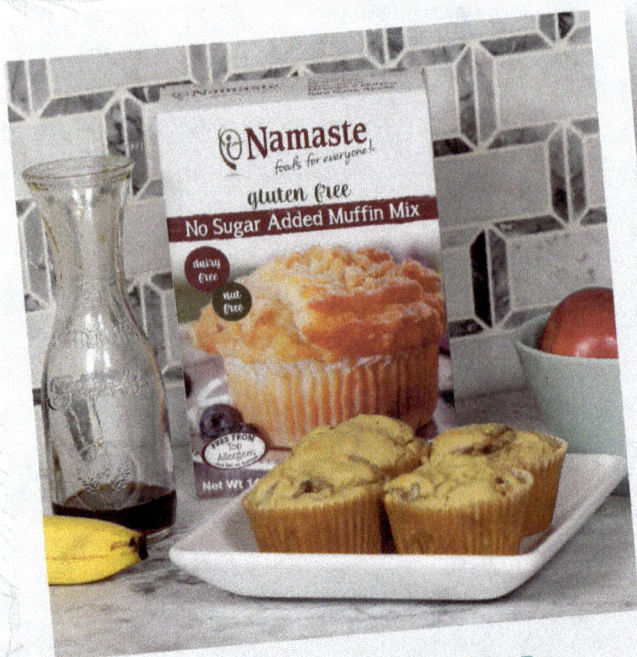

GLUTEN FREE!

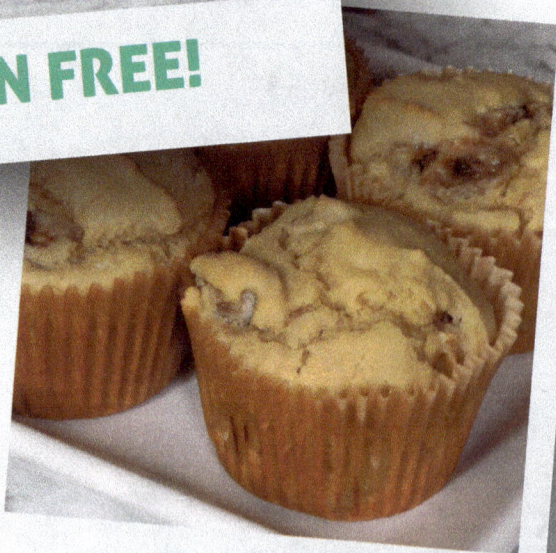

MUFFINS!

BANANA APPLE MUFFINS

INGREDIENTS

- 1 box Namaste No Sugar Muffin Mix and ingredients
- 1 Apple, peeled and diced
- 1 Banana, diced
- 1/4 Cup Maple Syrup

DIRECTIONS

Follow instructions on box stirring in apple and banana.
Bake as instructed in muffin wrappers.

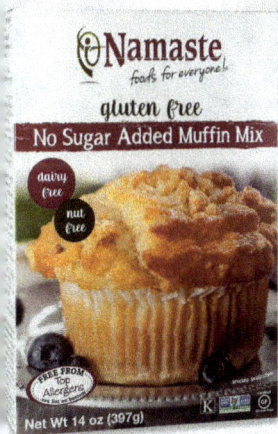

WHY NAMASTE

Namaste mixes are super easy and quick, especially for the weekend when you want a little treat. I love Namaste mixes because they are more than gluten free. They are a female owned company started by a mom who had a child with allergies. The mixes are top 8 free and can be measured out to make smaller batches. Many times we use half a box and save the remaining mix for another baking weekend. This helps us not overindulge.

BUY NAMASTE MUFFIN MIX

tinyurl.com/gfmommuffins

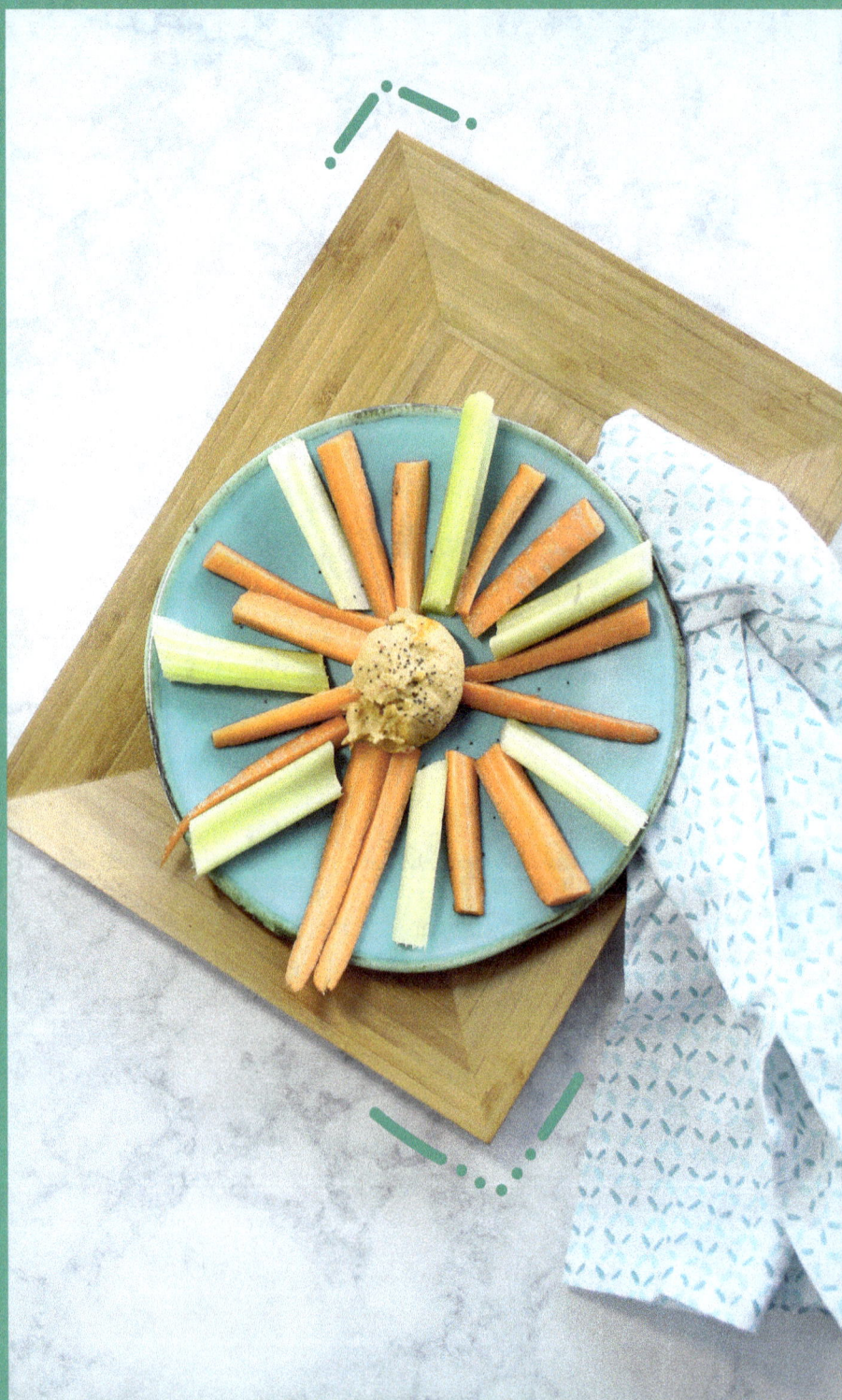

CARROTS AND ROASTED RED PEPPER HUMMUS

INGREDIENTS

- 1/2 Cup Baby Carrots
- 16 Oz Can Garbanzo Beans
- 1 Red Bell Pepper
- 1 Tbsp Red Onion, chopped
- 1 Clove Garlic, minced
- 1 Tbps Tahini
- 1 Lemon, juiced
- 2 Tbsp Olive Oil
- 1/2 Tsp Honey
- 1/2 Tsp Sriracha
- 1/2 Tsp Ground Cumin
- 1/2 Tsp Himalayan Salt

DIRECTIONS

- Drain and rinse the garbanzo beans. Roast the red bell pepper in broiler until grilled. Peel and seed the bell pepper. Combine all ingredients in a blender or food processor and process until smooth. You may have to stop and stir and/or scrape down sides a few times.
- Serve with carrots. Store leftover hummus in covered container in fridge for the rest of the week.

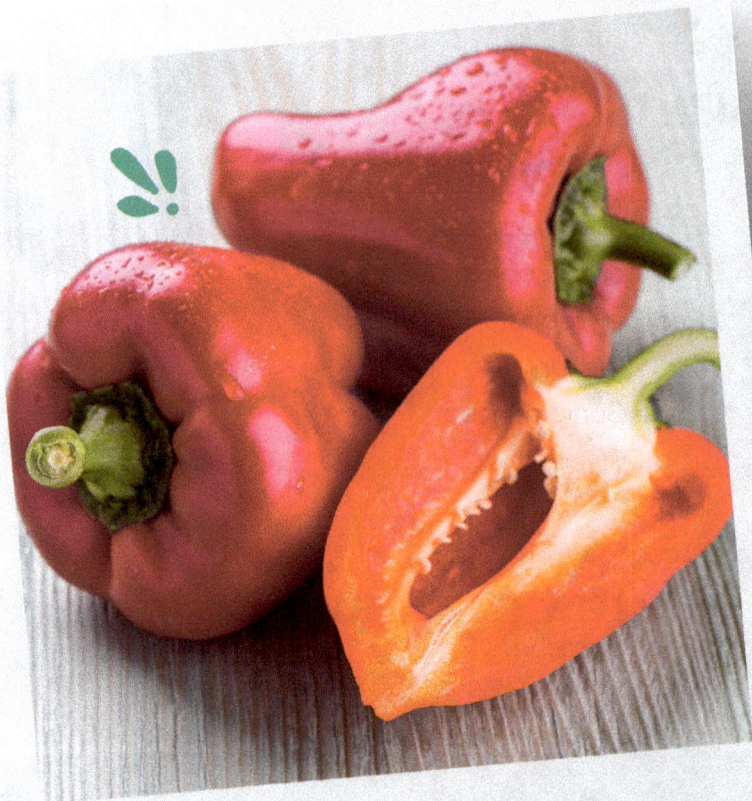

1 RED BELL PEPPER

GREEN PEPPER AND RED PEPPER HUMMUS

INGREDIENTS

- 1/2 Cup Green Pepper, sliced
- 16 Oz Can Garbanzo Beans
- 1 Red Bell Pepper
- 1 Tbsp Red Onion, chopped
- 1 Clove Garlic, minced
- 1 Tbsp Tahini
- 1 Lemon, juiced
- 2 Tbsp Olive Oil
- 1/2 Tsp Honey
- 1/2 Tsp Sriracha
- 1/2 Tsp Ground Cumin
- 1/2 Tsp Himalayan Salt

DIRECTIONS

- Drain and rinse the garbanzo beans. Roast the red bell pepper in broiler until grilled. Peel and seed the bell pepper. Combine all ingredients in a blender or food processor and process until smooth. You may have to stop and stir and/or scrape down sides a few times.
- Serve with green pepper. Store leftover hummus in covered container in fridge for the rest of the week.

#GFMOMCERTIFIED

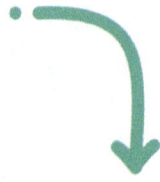

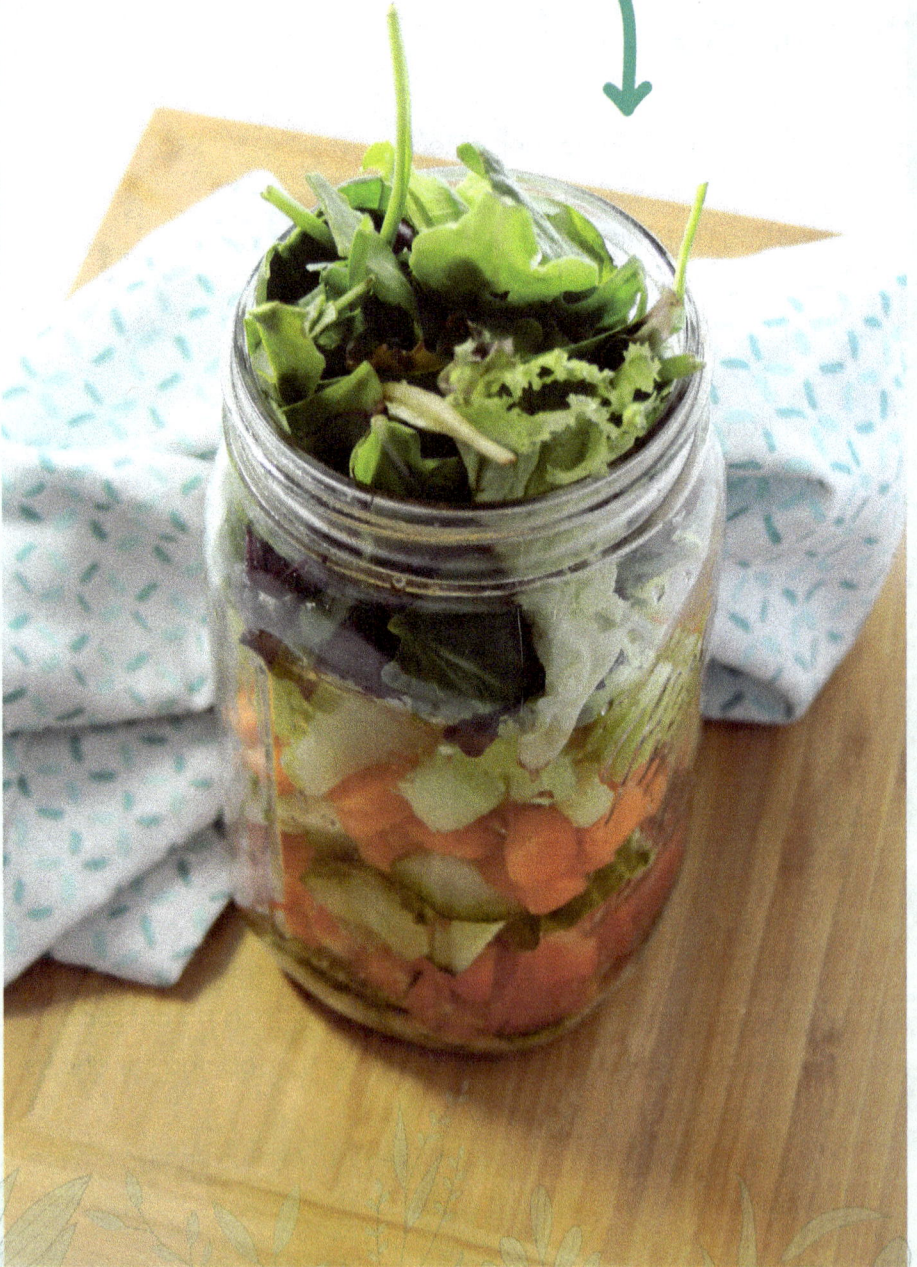

SALAD IN A JAR

INGREDIENTS

- 1 Cup Leafy Lettuce
- 1/2 Cup Spinach
- 1 Celery Stalk, finely chopped
- 1 Scallion, thinly sliced
- 1/2 Medium Cucumber, peeled and finely chopped
- 1 Red Bell Pepper, seeded and finely chopped
- 1 Small Carrot, peeled and finely chopped
- 1 Tbsp Olive Oil
- 1 Tbsp Apple Cider Vinegar
- 1 Tbsp Spicy Mustard
- 1 Garlic Clove, minced
- 1 Tbsp Fresh Lemon Juice
- 1/4 Tsp Himalayan Salt
- 1/4 Tsp Pepper

DIRECTIONS

- In a small bowl, combine olive oil, apple cider vinegar, spicy mustard, garlic, lemon juice, salt and pepper. In a widemouth Ball or Mason jar pour in dressing. Add carrots, red bell peppers, cucumber, celery and scallion. Top with spinach and lettuce. Screw on lid. Do not shake until ready to eat. You can store in fridge up to 3 days. The layered salad will stay fresh when air tight.

"LET FOOD BE THY MEDICINE, THY MEDICINE SHALL BE THY FOOD."

– HIPPOCRATES

SOUTHWEST TURBO SALAD

INGREDIENTS

- 1/2 Cup Baby Carrots
- 16 Oz Can Garbanzo Beans
- 1 Red Bell Pepper
- 1 Tbsp Red Onion, chopped
- 1 Clove Garlic, minced
- 1 Tbps Tahini
- 1 Lemon, juiced
- 2 Tbsp Olive Oil
- 1/2 Tsp Honey
- 1/2 Tsp Sriracha
- 1/2 Tsp Ground Cumin
- 1/2 Tsp Himalayan Salt

DIRECTIONS

- Drain and rinse the garbanzo beans. Roast the red bell pepper in broiler until grilled. Peel and seed the bell pepper. Combine all ingredients in a blender or food processor and process until smooth. You may have to stop and stir and/or scrape down sides a few times.
- Serve with carrots. Store leftover hummus in covered container in fridge for the rest of the week.

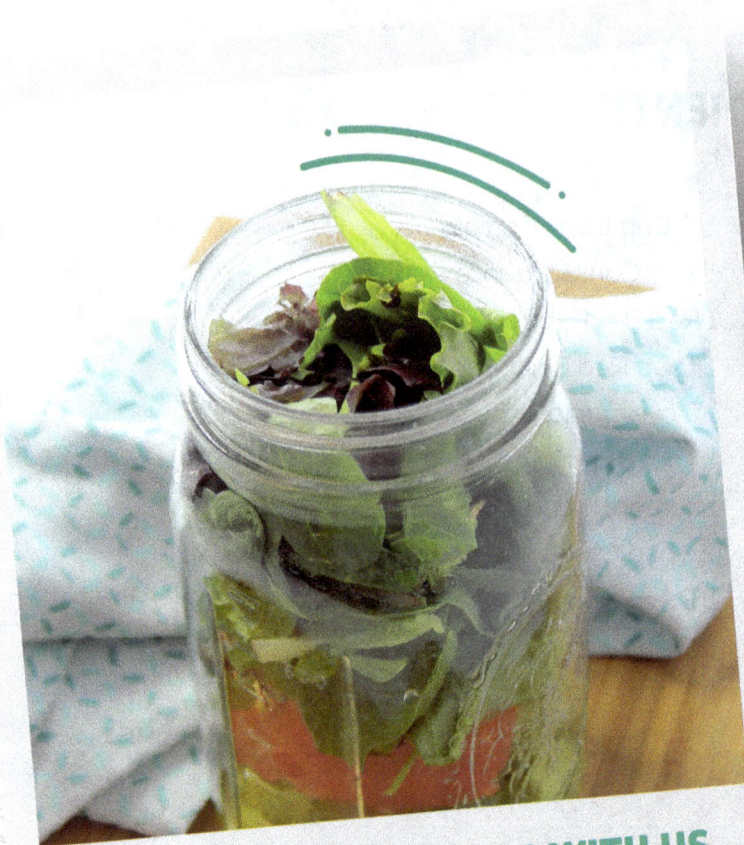

SHARE YOUR CREATIONS WITH US

#GFMOMCERTIFIED

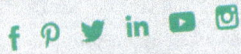

LITTLE ITALY SALAD IN A JAR

INGREDIENTS

- 1/2 Cup Leafy Lettuce
- 1/2 Cup Spinach
- 1/2 Avocado, thinly sliced
- 1/2 Cucumber, thinly sliced
- 1 Medium Tomato, thinly sliced
- 1 Pepperoncini, sliced
- 1 Tbsp Olive Oil
- 1 Tbsp Apple Cider Vinegar
- 1 Garlic Clove, minced
- 1 Tbsp Fresh Lemon Juice
- 1/4 Tsp Himalayan Salt
- 1/4 Tsp Pepper

DIRECTIONS

- In small bowl combine olive oil, apple cider vinegar, garlic, lemon juice, salt and pepper. In a wide-mouth Ball or Mason jar pour in dressing. Add avocado, cucumber, tomato and pepperoncini. Top with spinach and lettuce. Screw on lid. Do not shake until ready to eat. You can store in fridge up to 3 days. The layered salad will stay fresh when air tight.

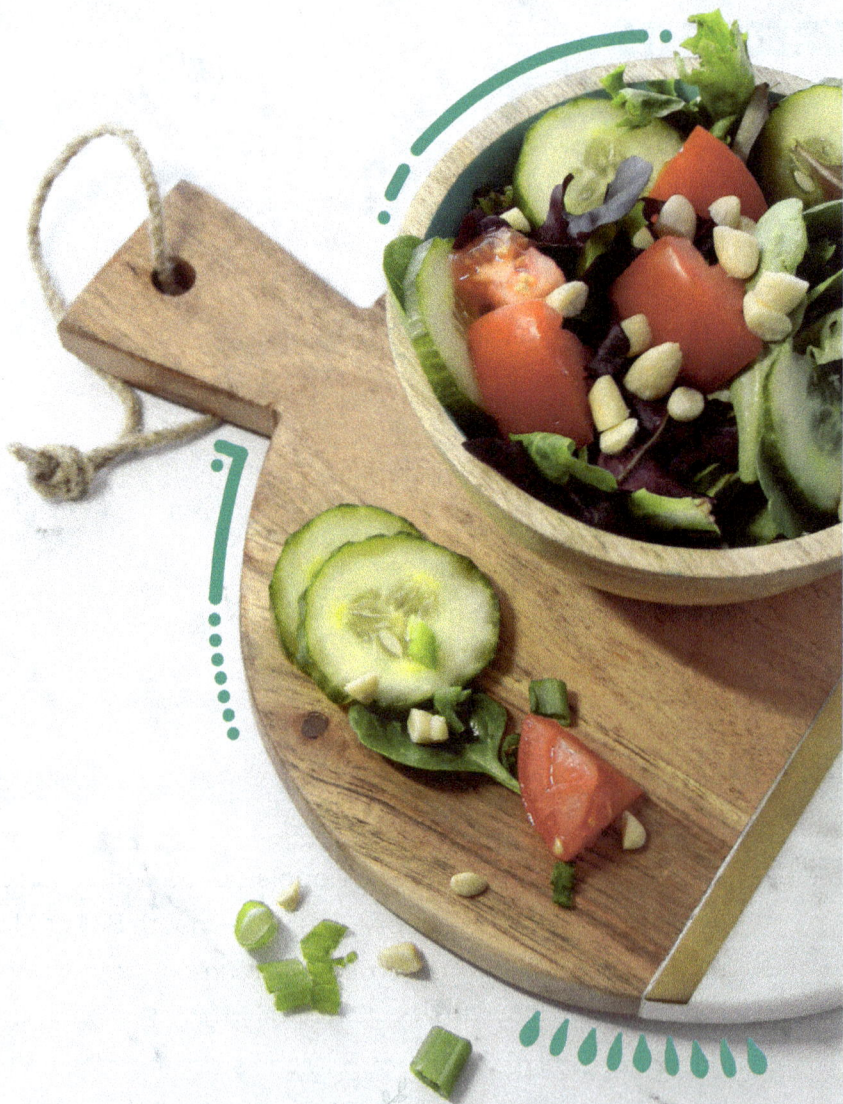

MIXED GREEN SALAD WITH ALMONDS

INGREDIENTS

- 1/2 Cup Mixed Salad Greens
- 1/2 Medium Tomato, diced
- 1/4 Cucumber, sliced
- 1/4 Cup Almond Slivers
- 1 and 1/2 Tsp Balsamic Vinegar

DIRECTIONS

- Combine all ingredients and drizzle with vinegar. Toss gently to blend.

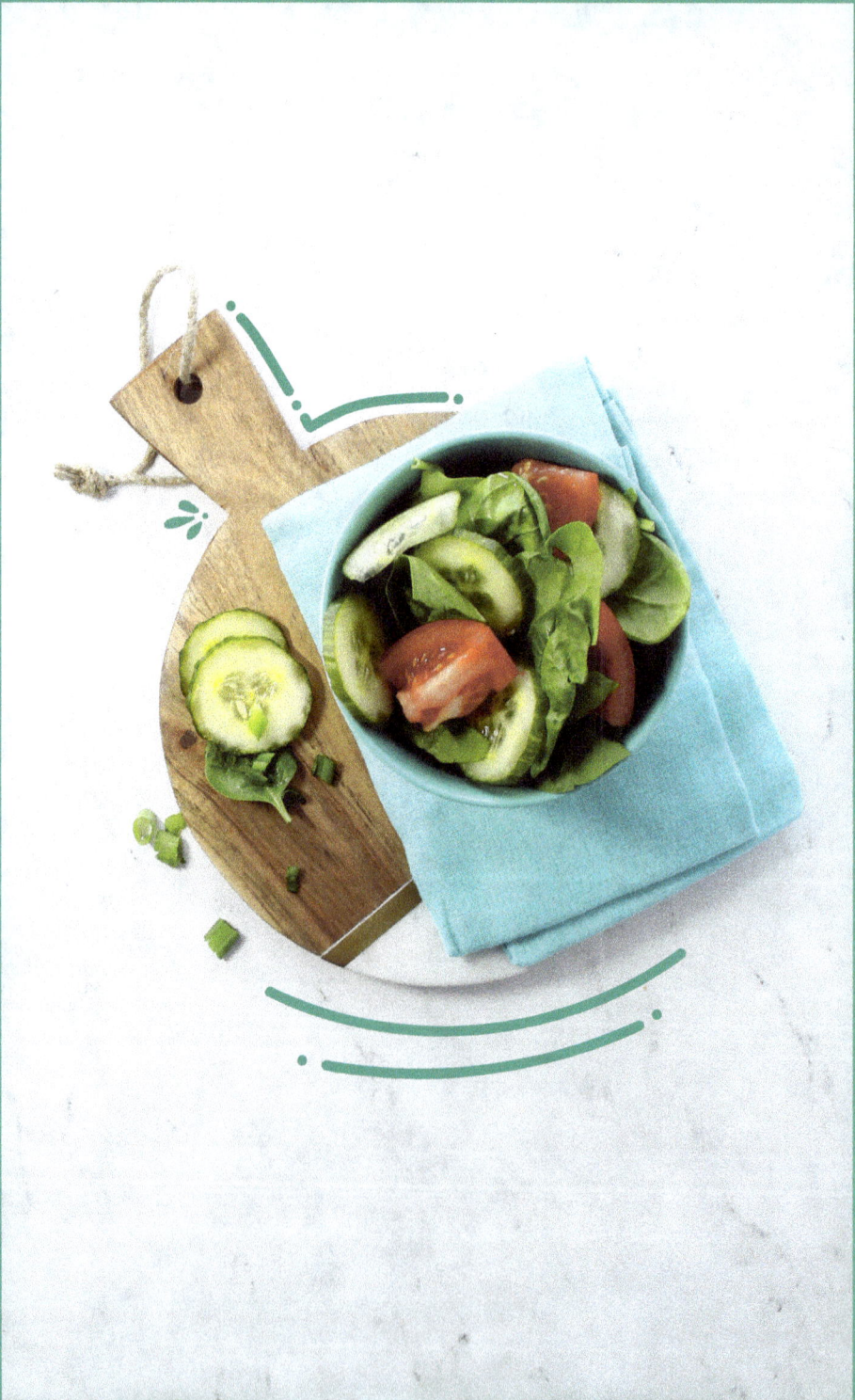

SIMPLE SPINACH SALAD

INGREDIENTS

- 4 Cups Fresh Spinach
- 1 Medium Tomato, cut into wedges
- 1/2 Cucumber, sliced
- 1 and 1/2 Tsp Olive Oil
- 1 and 1/2 Tsp Balsamic Vinegar

DIRECTIONS

- Combine spinach, tomato and cucumber in a large serving bowl. Drizzle with oil and vinegar; toss gently to blend.

VEGGIE STIR-FRY

INGREDIENTS

- 2 Tbsp Coconut Oil
- 1 Tbsp Sesame Oil
- 1 Tsp Crushed Red Pepper Flakes
- 2 Cups Broccoli Florets
- 1 Red Bell Pepper, sliced thinly
- 1 Cup Snap Peas
- 2 Cups Carrots, peeled and sliced thinly
- 2 Cups Green Beans
- 5 Garlic Cloves, minced
- 1 Tbsp Fresh Ginger, grated
- 4 Tbsp Rice Vinegar
- 2 Tbsp Liquid Aminos or San J Tamari
- 2 Tbsp Raw Honey
- 1/4 Cup Slivered Almonds
- 1 Cup Bib Lettuce for Wraps

DIRECTIONS

- In large skillet over medium-high heat, add oils and red pepper flakes. Add veggies and stir continuously until veggies are crisp-tender. Add garlic and ginger, and cook 1 minute. In a small bowl whisk together vinegar, aminos and honey. Add to skillet, cook 2-3 minutes. Remove from heat, and sprinkle with almonds. Serve wrapped in lettuce.

ROASTED CHICKEN BITES AND VEGGIES

INGREDIENTS

- 2 Boneless Skinless Chicken Breasts, cut into chunks
- Vegan - Portabella Mushrooms
- 2 Zucchinis, cubed
- 1 Green Pepper, rough chopped
- 1 Red Pepper, rough chopped
- 1 Red Onion, peeled and chopped
- 1 Tsp Himalayan Salt
- 1/2 Tsp Pepper
- 1/2 Tsp Chili Powder
- 2 Garlic Cloves, minced
- 1 Tbsp Grapeseed Oil

DIRECTIONS

- Preheat oven to 450°. Mix all ingrdients in large bowl and toss to coat. Lay mixture in single layer on a baking sheet lined with parchment paper or silpat mat. Cook for 20 minutes. Rotate and cook for additional 20 minutes or until edges are crispy and begin to brown slightly.

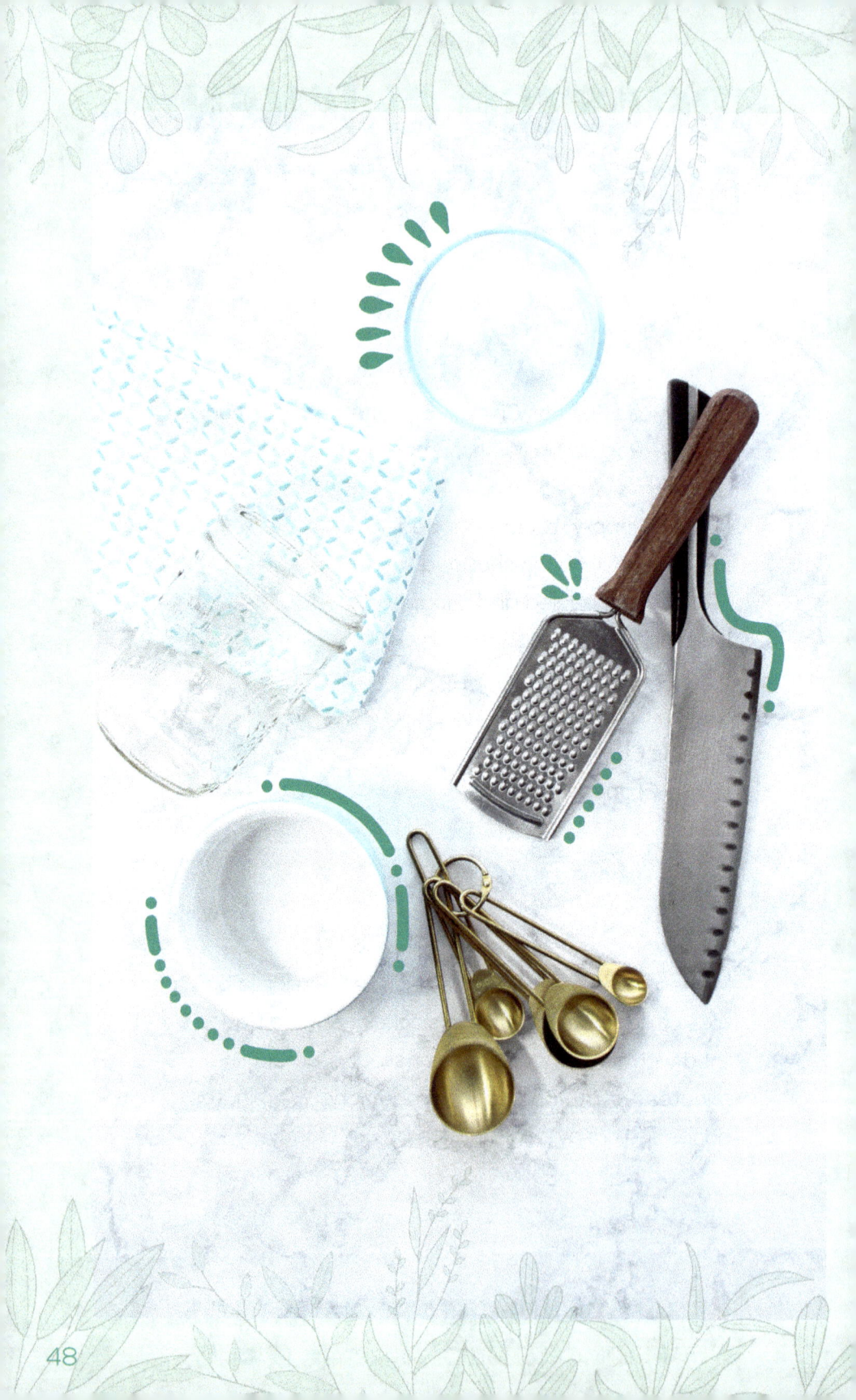

VEGGIE CURRY OVER SWEET POTATO

INGREDIENTS

- 2 Medium Red Onions, sliced long
- 3 Cloves Garlic, shelled
- 1 Inch Ginger, chopped
- 4 Large Tomatoes, chopped
- 1 Can Chickpeas, drained
- 2 Tbsp Coconut Oil
- 1 Tsp Turmeric
- 1 Tsp Red Chili Powder
- 1/2 Tsp Himalayan Salt
- 2 Tsp Chole Masala
- 1/2 Cup Coconut Milk
- 2 Large Sweet Potato

DIRECTIONS

- Heat oven to 400° and bake sweet potato until soft. Once sweet potato is in the oven begin your curry. Puree, in food processor or blender, red onion, garlic and ginger until it forms a thick paste. Heat coconut oil in a large skillet. Once melted add onion paste. Fry onion mixture until it starts to brown. Add tomatoes and cook till they begin to soften, about 5 minutes, stirring often. Add turmeric, red chili powder and salt. Mix well. Cook for 3 minutes. Add chole masala * and mix together. Then add chickpeas and stir. Slowly stir in coconut milk and lower heat to simmer. Stir occasionally and continue to simmer until the sweet potato is done. Approximately 40 minutes.
- *chickpeas are called chole in hindi

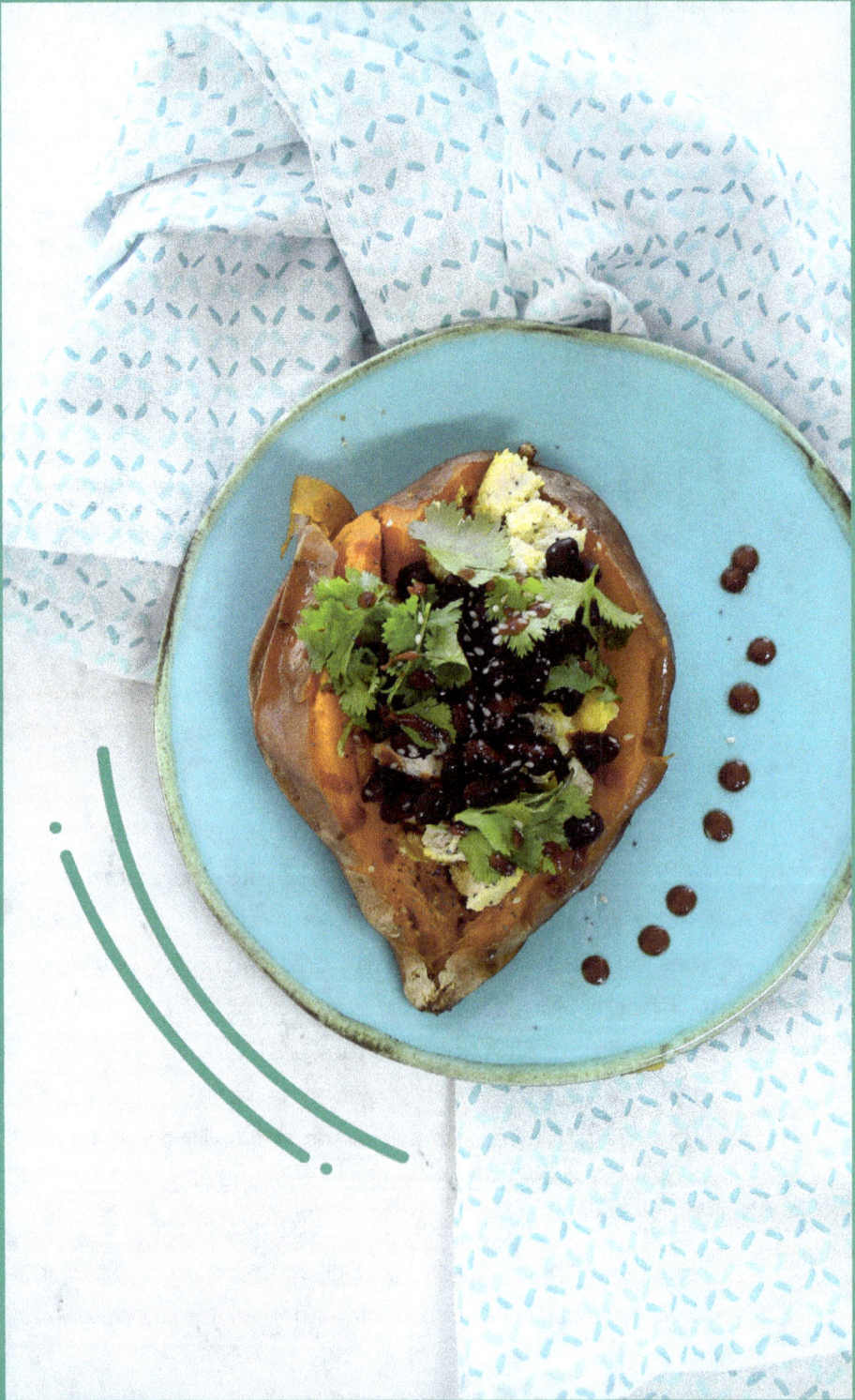

BAKED STUFFED SWEET POTATO

INGREDIENTS

- 2 Small Sweet Potatoes, pierced with a fork several times
- 1 and 1/2 Cups Shredded Chicken or Tofu
- 1/2 Cup Black Beans
- 2 Tsp Olive Oil
- 1/2 Tsp Ground Cumin
- 1/2 Tsp Ground Coriander
- 1/4 Tsp Himalayan Salt
- 2 Tbsp Cilantro, chopped

DIRECTIONS

- Preheat oven to 400°. Bake sweet potatoes for 40 minutes or until tender. Cut sweet potatoes almost in half lengthwise.
- While sweet potatoes are baking, combine chicken, beans, oil, cumin, coriander and salt in a small pan. Cook over medium heat stirring constantly for 5 minutes.
- Top sweet potatoes evenly with chicken mixture. Sprinkle with cilantro.

PIZZA AND SALAD

INGREDIENTS

- 1 Cup Potato Starch
- 1/4 Cup Coconut Flour
- 1 Tsp Baking Powder
- 1/2 Cup Water
- 1/4 Cup Olive Oil
- 1 Tsp Garlic, Minced
- 1 Tsp Oregano
- 1 Tsp Himalayan Salt
- 1 Tbsp Apple Cider Vinegar + Coconut Milk to make 1/4 cup total
- 1/4 Cup Tomato Sauce or Organic Pizza Sauce
- 1 Red Onion, thinly sliced
- 1 Green Pepper, thinly sliced
- 1/2 Cup Spinach Leaves, torn
- Pepperoni slices (optional)

DIRECTIONS

- Preheat oven to 450°. Line a cookie sheet or baking stone with parchment paper. Place the pan in the oven to get warm. In a large bowl, mix coconut flour, potato starch, baking powder and Himalayan salt. Stir in the warm water and olive oil and mix until combined. Let this set for 3-5 minutes, it will thicken up as the coconut flour absorbs the liquid. Add vinegar/milk mixture and mix together with garlic and oregano.

Remove the baking sheet from the oven and pour the flat bread dough on to the parchment paper. Spread around.

Cook for 12 minutes in the oven until the edges start to brown. Remove, top with tomato sauce, red onion, green pepper, spinach leaves and pepperoni. Bake for 10 more minutes.

Serve with Salad made with leftover veggies from the week! Enjoy!

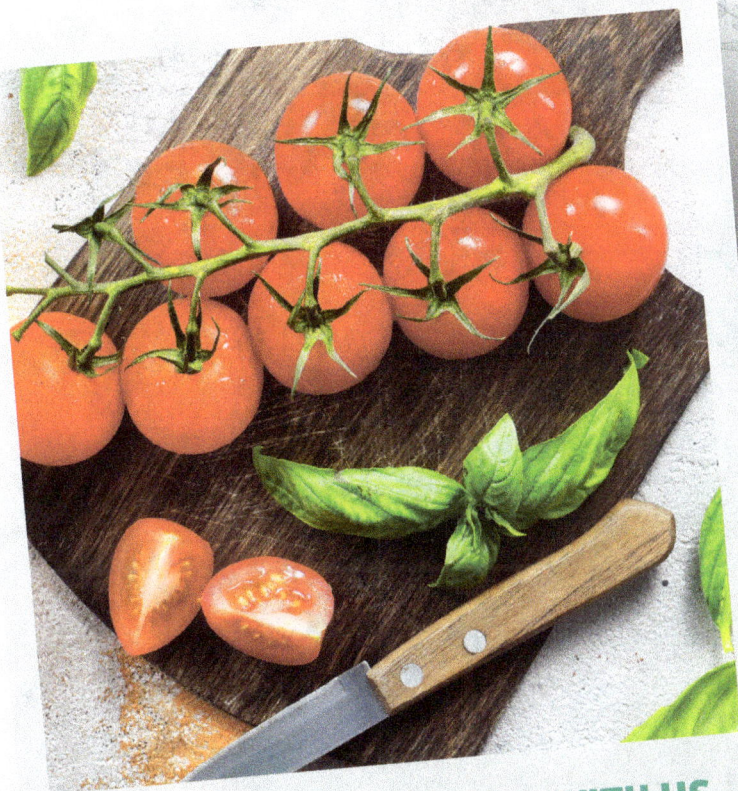

SHARE YOUR CREATIONS WITH US

#GFMOMCERTIFIED

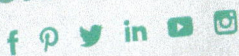

WORKOUT EXERCISES

SQUATS

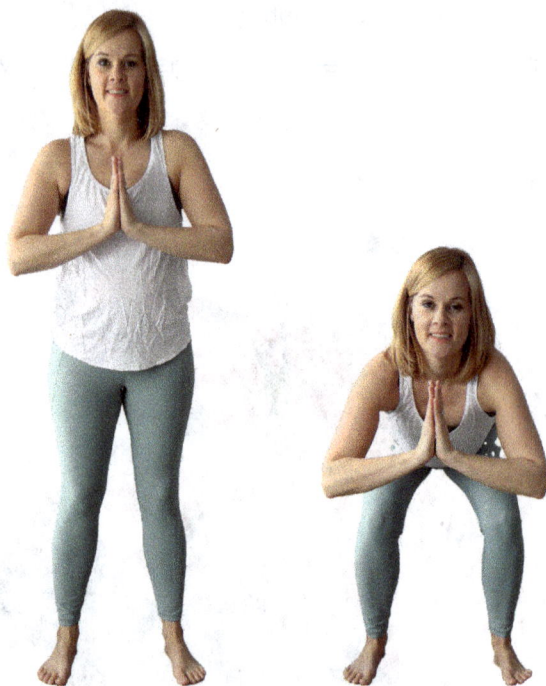

SEATED HIP ROTATION

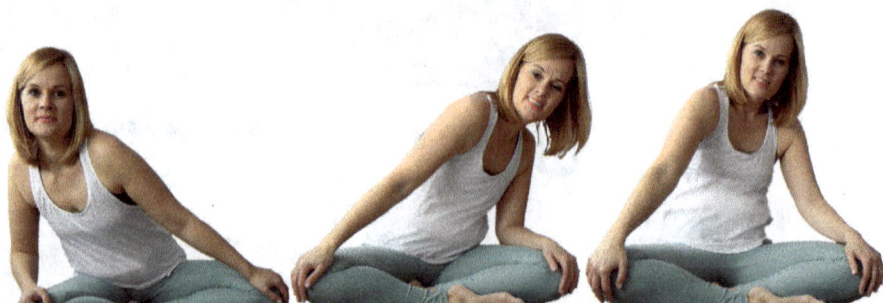

TORSO TWIST

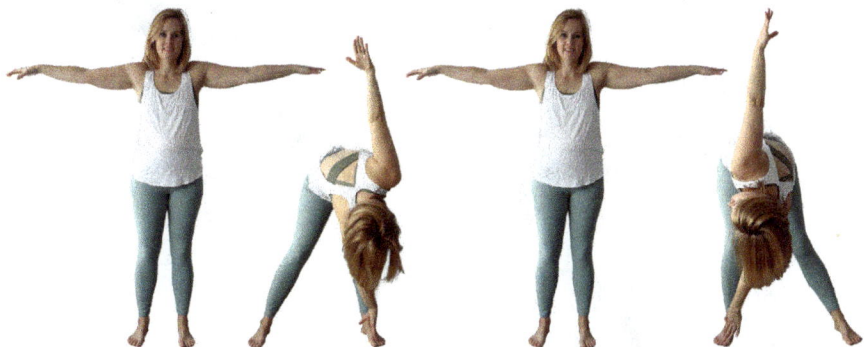

SWEEPS

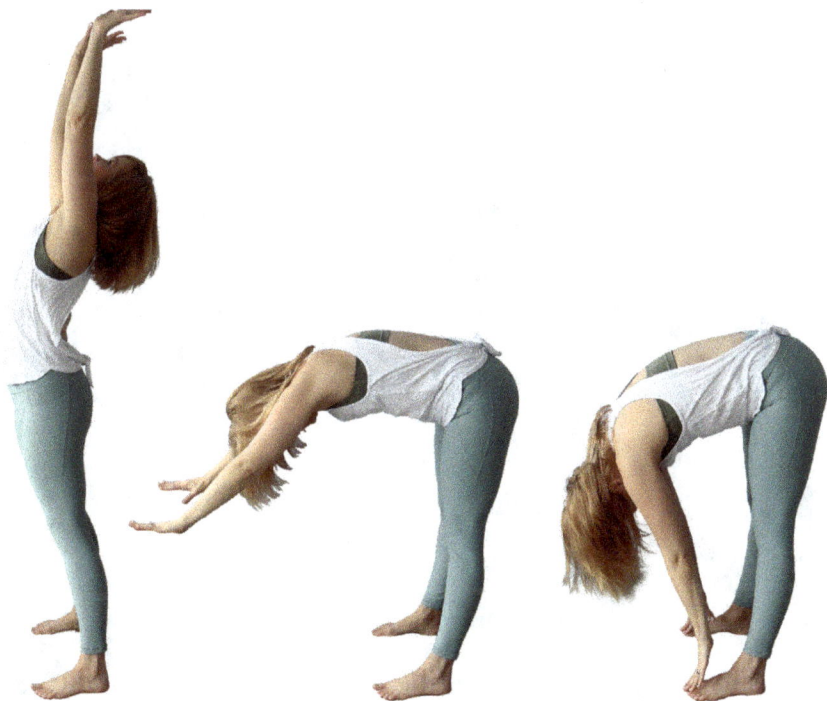

JOURNAL EXERCISES

Draw 2 Stick People and fill in, with words, for the questions below.

- Q: Person 1 – How my body feels right now

- Q: Person 2 – How I'd love my body to feel

Write 100 things you are grateful for in your life.

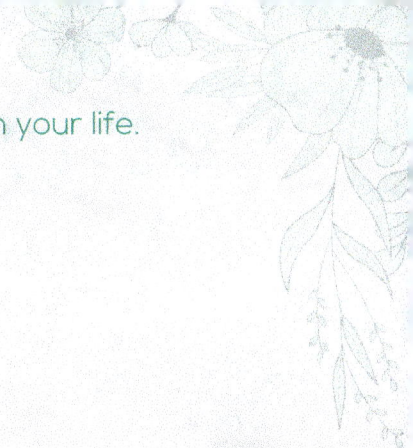

DETOX MUST-HAVES

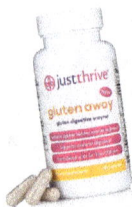

JUST THRIVE GLUTEN AWAY™

Gluten Away™ is a unique blend of powerful digestive enzymes and probiotics designed t support optimal gluten digestion and protec against hidden sources of gluten. It contains a proprietary blend of two spore-based probiotics and Sacchromyces Boulardii, as w as four specific enzymes and Betaine HCL.

USE CODE GFMOM FOR 15% OFF
JUSTTHRIVEHEALTH.COM

NAMASTE GLUTEN-FREE PERFECT FLOUR BLEND

Namaste Foods is a women-owned, family-operated maker of exceptionally tasty food that is better for you than the run-of-the mill choices on most grocery store shelves. Our delicious Namaste Gluten-free Perfect Flour Blend is free from the Top 8 allergens making it the safe for people challenged by food allergies and sensitivities.

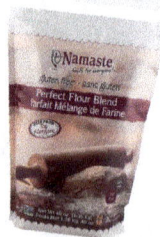

TINYURL.COM/GFMOMNAMASTE

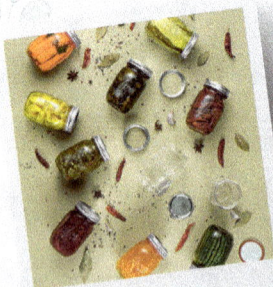

6 PACK, 16 OZ MASON JARS

Superior Lid-Mason jars are self-sealing for airtight and leak proof perfection. The metal is lined with plastisol, avoiding rust and decay Food contained will last longer and taste fresher. Dishwasher safe.

TINYURL.COM/GFMOMJAR

IMPERFECT FOODS

Delivering groceries on a mission to fight food waste and build a better food system for everyone. Head to our website to see if we deliver to you!

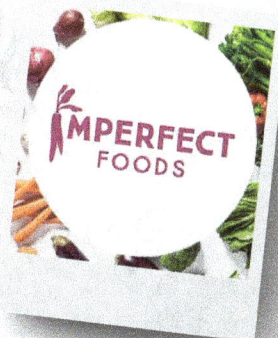

$10 OFF 1ST ORDER

TINYURL.COM/GFMOMIMPERFECT

THE SOULFULL PROJECT INSTANT OATMEAL MULTI-SERVE BAG

Ready in minutes with either hot water or your favorite milk, a healthy blend of whole grain rye, whole oats, barley and toasted red quinoa takes your everyday oatmeal experience to a whole new level. Non-GMO Project Verified, Certified Vegan, and Whole Grain Stamp Approved. Each serving is packed with 4 grams of protein and 6 grams of fiber.

TINYURL.COM/GFMOMSOULFULL

THE ALMOND COW PLANT-BASED STARTER SET

Use any nut, seed, or grain to make homemade plant-based milk in moments. Makes 5-6 cups of fresh milk at the touch of a button. No straining. No mess. Easy cleanup. Just the way it should be!

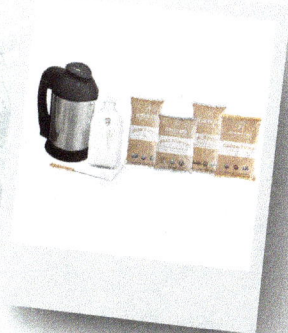

USE THE LINK BELOW FOR $10 OFF

TINYURL.COM/GFMOMALMONDCOW

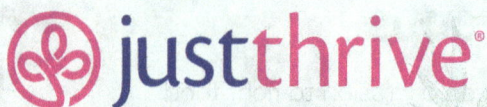

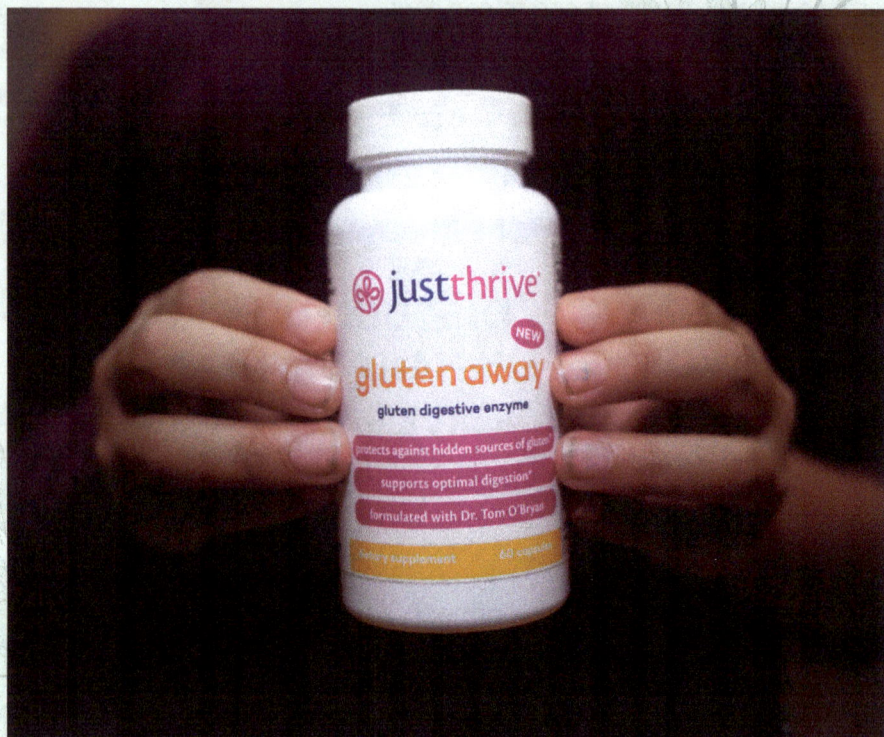

JUST THRIVE GLUTEN AWAY™

Gluten Away™ is a unique blend of powerful digestive enzymes and probiotics designed to support optimal gluten digestion and protect against hidden sources of gluten. It contains a proprietary blend of two spore-based probiotics and Sacchromyces Boulardii, as well as four specific enzymes and Betaine HCL.

Use the code GFMOM to get 15% off your order. justthrivehealth.com

WEEK 2

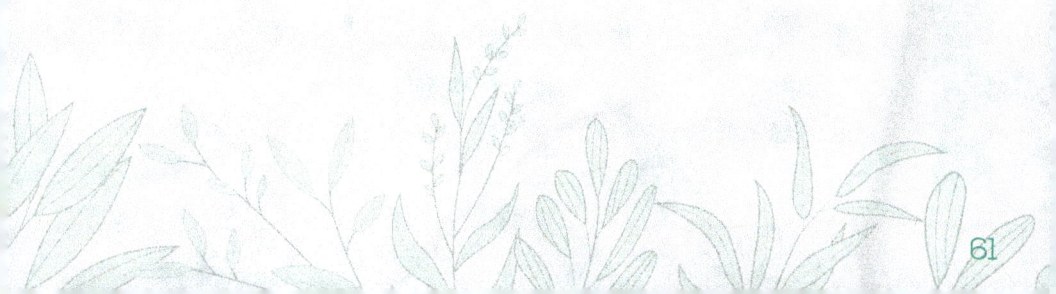

WEEK 2 MENU

	MON	TUE	WED	THU	FRI
BREAKFAST	Colada Smoothie	Strawberry Banana Smoothie	Strawberry Banana Smoothie	Chocolate Banana Almond Smoothie	Chocolate Banana Almond Smoothie
AM SNACK	Berry Mix Salad	Berry Mix Salad	Berry Mix Salad	Berry Mix Salad	Green Apple and Almond Butter
LUNCH	Salad in a Jar	Mediterranean Chicken Salad	Simple Spinach Salad	Southwest Turbo Salad	Leftover Chili with Side Salad
PM SNACK	Melon Refresh	Melon Refresh	Melon Refresh	Carrots and Roasted Red Hummus	Carrots and Roasted Red Hummus
DINNER	Mediterranean Chicken Salad	Chicken and Veggie Tacos in Lettuce Wraps	Veggie Curry Over Sweet Potato	4 Bean Chili	Pizza and Salad

✓	GROCERY LIST	QTY
☐	Packages of Strawberries (Freeze 1)	2
☐	Packages of Raspberries (Freeze 1)	2
☐	Package of Blackberries	1
☐	Package of Blueberries	1
☐	Pineapple	1
☐	Watermelon	1
☐	Cantaloupe	1
☐	Honeydew	1
☐	Oranges	4
☐	Lemons	4
☐	Granny Smith Apples	3
☐	Bundle of Spotted Bananas	1
☐	Heads of Leaf Lettuce	2
☐	Mixed Greens	1
☐	Bunches of Spinach	2
☐	Celery Packages	1
☐	Cucumbers	3
☐	Red Bell Peppers	3
☐	Green Bell Peppers	3

✓	GROCERY LIST	QTY
☐	Yellow Bell Pepper	1
☐	Red Onions	5
☐	Spanish Onions	2
☐	Sweet Potatoes	2
☐	Carrots	2
☐	Baby Carrots	1
☐	Fresh Ginger	1
☐	Garlic Bulbs	2
☐	Tomatoes	14
☐	Cherry Tomatoes	1
☐	Avocados	5
☐	Fresh Cilantro	1
☐	Fresh Basil	1
☐	Fresh Mint	1
☐	Fresh Parsley	1
☐	Organic Fermented Tofu	1
☐	Gallons of Coconut Milk	2.5
☐	Egg (Optional)	1
☐	Ground Flax	1

✓	GROCERY LIST	QTY
☐	Almond Butter	1
☐	Sliced Almonds	1
☐	Chopped Walnuts	1
☐	Chicken Breasts	3
☐	lb of Ground Turkey	1
☐	lb of Sliced Pepperoni	1
☐	Cans of Chickpeas	3
☐	Cans of Black Beans	2
☐	Can of Kidney Beans	1
☐	Can of Great Northern Beans	1

PANTRY STAPLES

Potato Starch

Coconut Flour

Coconut Flakes (Raw)

Himalayan Salt

Pepper

Red Chili Powder

Oregano

Cacao

Onion Powder

Cayenne

Turmeric

Coriander

Chole Masala

Red Pepper Flakes

Aqua Fava (Bean Water)

Cumin

CONDIMENTS

Olive Oil	Balsamic Vinegar	Apple Cider Vinegar
Grapeseed Oil	Pesto	
Coconut Oil	Sriracha	Spicy Mustard (Non-GMO/Sugar Free)
Raw Honey	Louisiana Hot Sauce	
Tomato Sauce		

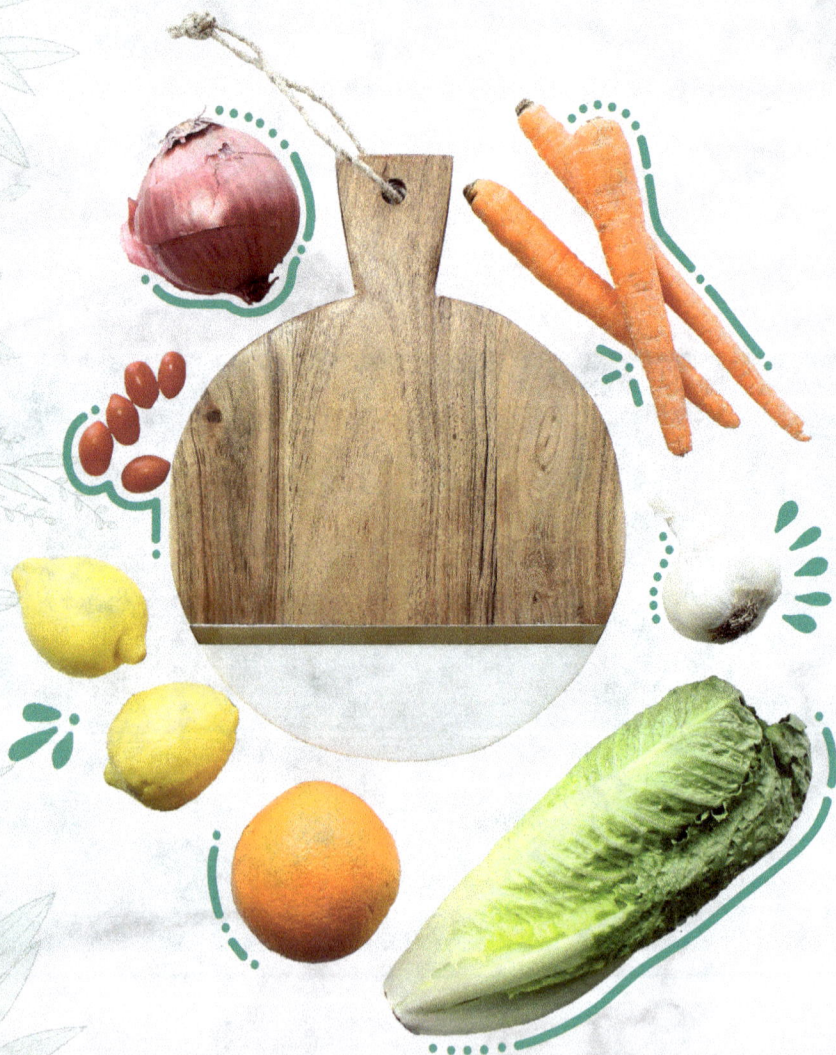

YOU'RE DOING GREAT
YOU'RE DOING GREAT
YOU'RE DOING GREAT
YOU'RE DOING GREAT
YOU'RE DOING GREAT

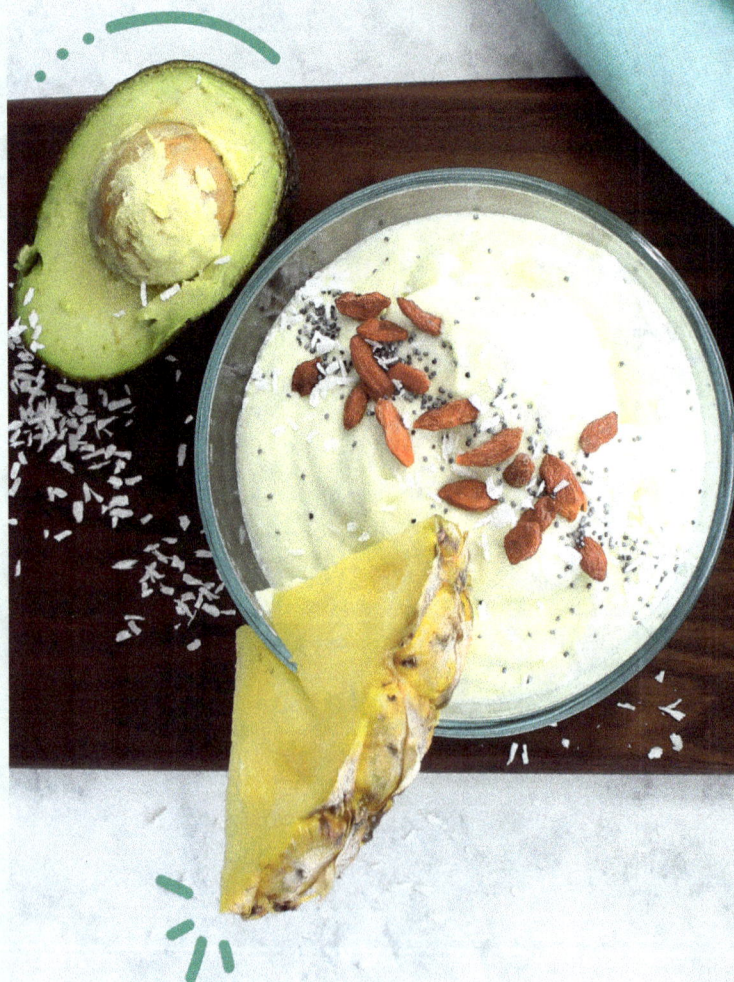

COLADA SMOOTHIE

INGREDIENTS

- 1 Cup Coconut Milk
- 1/2 Cup Pineapple, cubed
- 1/2 Avocado
- 2 Tbsp Coconut Flakes, raw
- 1 Small Lime, juiced
- 1 Tsp Lime Zest

DIRECTIONS

- Place all ingredients in blender and blend until creamy. The more ice or frozen berries, the thicker it gets.

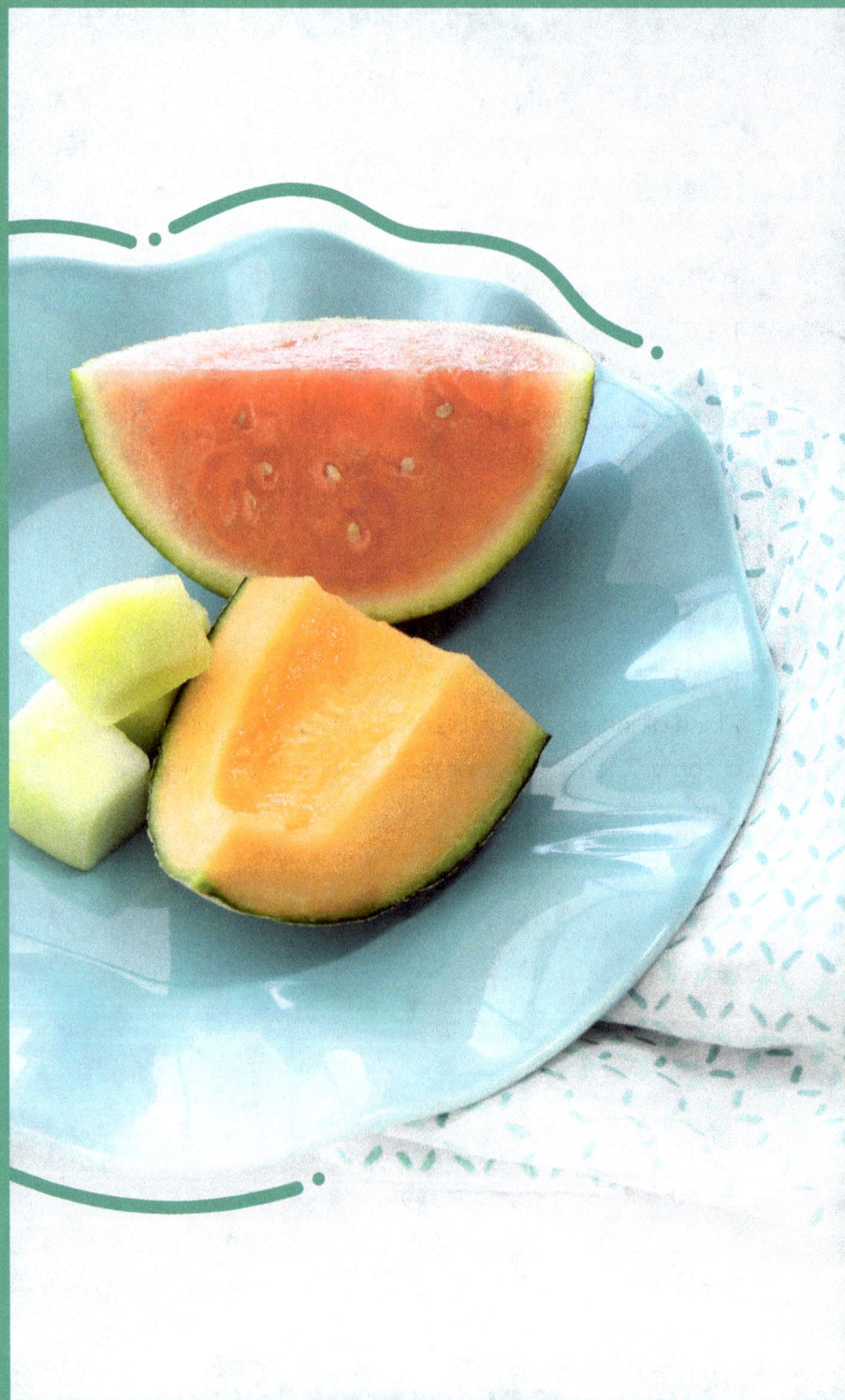

MELON REFRESH

INGREDIENTS

- 1 Cup Watermelon, cubed
- 1/2 Cup Cantaloupe, cubed
- 1/2 Cup Honeydew Melon, cubed
- 1 Tbsp Walnuts, chopped
- Fresh Mint Leaves (optional)

DIRECTIONS

- Combine all ingredients and mix well. Top with mint if desired.
- Make up a large bowl and have it ready for the week.

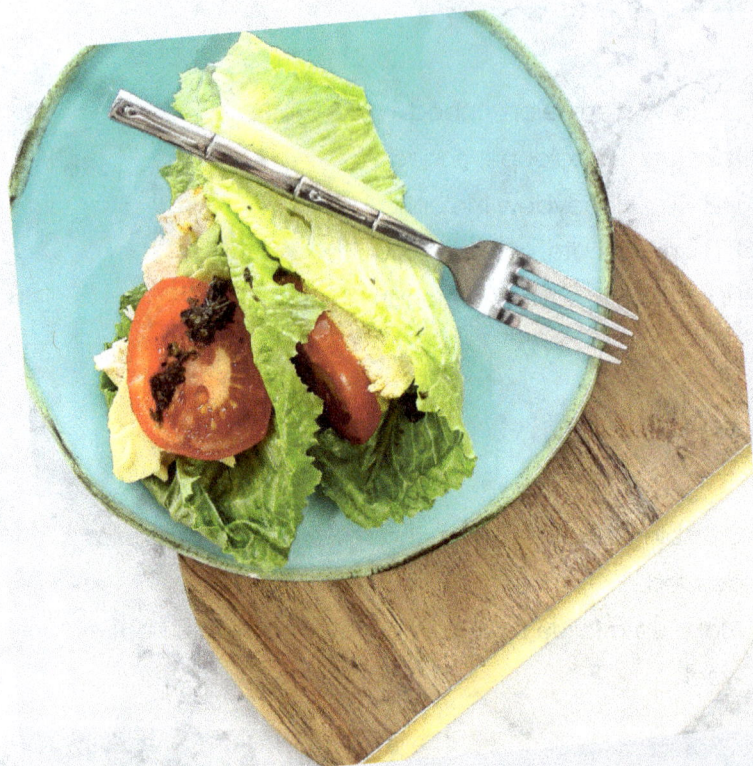

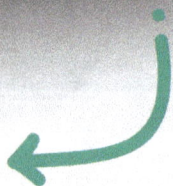 **TASTY!**

MEDITERRANEAN CHICKEN SALAD

NGREDIENTS

- 1 4oz Chicken Breast, cut into 1 inch pieces (Replace with mushrooms for Vegan)
- 1 Tbsp and 1 tsp Extra Virgin Olive Oil
- 1 Tsp Balsamic Vinegar
- 2 Tbsp Fresh Lemon
- 1 Garlic Clove, minced
- Dash of Himalayan Salt
- Dash of Black Pepper
- 1 Cucumber
- 6 Cherry Tomatoes, halved
- 1/4 Cup Fresh Parsley, torn
- 1 Scallion, thinly sliced
- 1 Cup Baby Spinach

IRECTIONS

- Toss chicken with 1 tsp oil, 1 Tbsp lemon juice, garlic, salt and pepper. In medium skillet cook chicken 7-8 minutes over medium-high heat or until cooked through. In bowl combine cucumber, tomato, parsley, scallion, spinach, chicken; toss with 1 Tbsp lemon juice, 1 Tbsp oil, 1 tsp balsamic vinegar. Season with Himalayan salt and pepper, to taste.

4 BEAN CHILI

INGREDIENTS

- 1 lb Ground Beef or Turkey
- 1 Medium Onion, chopped
- 1 Green Pepper, chopped
- 1 and 3/4 Cups Water
- 6 Large Tomatoes, chopped
- 1 Can Kidney Beans
- 1 Can Great Northern Beans
- 1 Can Garbanzo Beans
- 1 Can Black Beans
- 1 Tbsp Cacao Powder
- 2 Tsp Louisiana Hot Sauce
- 1/2 Tsp Black Pepper
- 1/2 Tsp Chili Powder
- 2 Cloves Garlic, minced
- 1/8 Tsp Cayenne Pepper

DIRECTIONS

- In a dutch oven or large pot cook meat, onion and green pepper until meat is no longer pink. Drain.
- Stir in all remaining ingredients. Bring to a boil, reduce heat and simmer for at least 30 minutes.
- You can mix all ingredients into a crock pot and cook for 8 hours on low.

CHICKEN AND VEGGIE TACOS IN LETTUCE WRAPS

INGREDIENTS

- 2 Chicken Breasts, Sliced
- 1 Tsp Cumin
- 1 Tsp Chili Powder
- 1/8 Tsp Himalayan Salt
- 1/8 Tsp Black Pepper
- 1/8 Tsp Red Pepper Flakes
- 1/2 Tsp Garlic Powder
- 1/2 Tsp Onion Powder
- 2 Tbsp Olive Oil
- 1/2 Cup Red Bell Pepper
- 1/2 Cup Yellow Bell Pepper
- 1/2 Cup Green Bell Pepper
- 1/2 Cup Red Onion
- 1 Lime
- Lettuce for Wraps or 1 Package Potapas Tortillas

DIRECTIONS

- Slice the chicken into 1/4 inch strips and place into a zipper bag or bowl. Add the spices and 1 tbs olive oil. Seal and shake to coat the meat. Place in the fridge while you prep vegetables.
- Clean and slice the peppers and onion into 1/4 inch strips.
- In a skillet, heat the remaining olive oil on high heat. Add the spiced chicken and the sliced vegetables. Reduce heat to medium and cook; stirring often until the vegetables begin to soften and the meat is cooked. Slice the lime and squeeze half of the lime over the meat. Stir well. Serve with lettuce wraps or Potapas Tortillas.

JOURNAL EXERCISES

Q: What are the areas that feel out of whack, hard to follow or crazy in your health?

Q: How can you help your health thrive?

EXERCISE MUST-HAVES

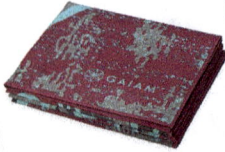

GAIAM FOLDABLE YOGA MAT

The Yoga Revolution is here. At Gaiam we know yoga. Gaiam's Foldable Yoga Mat is a 2mm thick, scored yoga mat that folds to a 10 inch x 12 inch compact square and easily fits into your carry-on or tote bag.

TINYURL.COM/GFMOMYOGAMAT

GAIAM DUMBBELLS HAND WEIGHTS

These durable cast-iron hand weights feature a neoprene shell that provides a comfortable non slip grip. The hexagonal shape keeps the weight from rolling while not in use and helps to prevent damage to floors. Ideal for beginners to advanced in a home gym or studio for muscle toning and weight training, cardio workouts, physical therapy and rehabilitation and more!

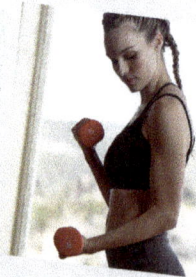

TINYURL.COM/GFMOMDUMBBELL

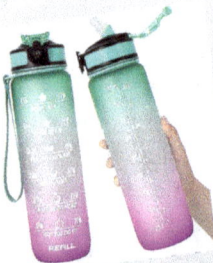

MOTIVATIONAL WATER BOTTL WITH TIME MARKER & STRAW

Designed with time marker and inspirational quotes, Fimibuke water bottle is perfect for helping you stay motivated to drink enough water throughout the day. Featured with translucent appearance and capacity scale helps you measure your daily intake of water easily and clearly.

TINYURL.COM/GFMOMBOTTLE

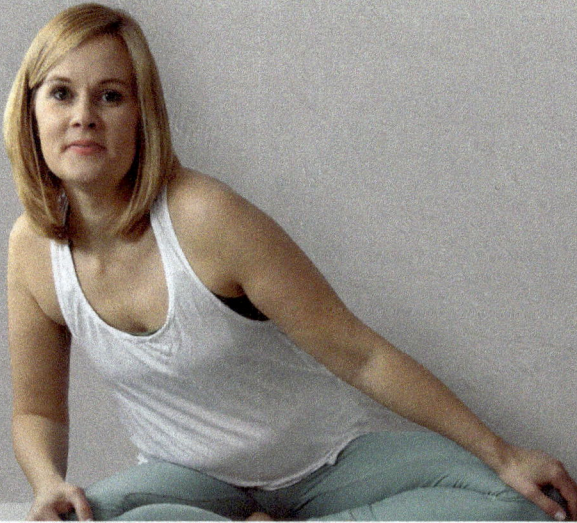

OLD NAVY

Get the newest looks at affordable prices in every style, size and color. Our family loves our new comfy and cozy activewear. Does your family love Old Navy as much as ours? Get your own healthy living gear by using our GF Mom Certified affiliate link below. Use #sayhi on Instagram @oldnavy to share your funnest, funniest, fashioniest Old Navy moments!

gap.igs4ds.net/kndEn

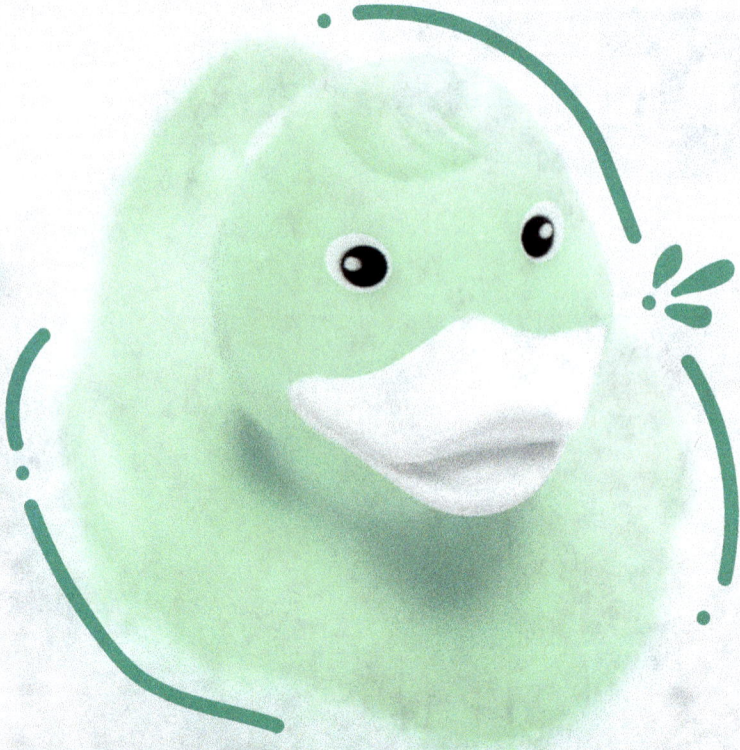

WHEN IN DOUBT TAKE A BATH.

-MAE WEST

WEEK 3

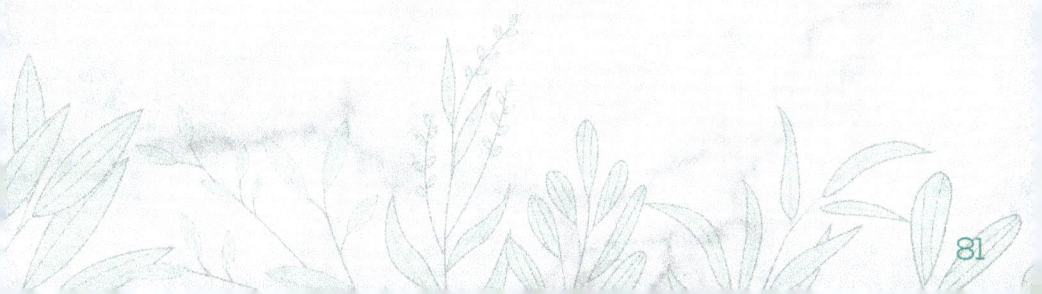

WEEK 3 MENU

	MON	TUE	WED	THU	FRI
BREAKFAST	Strawberry Banana Smoothie	Chocolate Banana Almond Smoothie	Strawberry Banana Smoothie	Strawberry Banana Smoothie	Strawberry Banana Smoothie
AM SNACK	Berry Mix Salad	Berry Mix Salad	Berry Mix Salad	Granola and Fresh Fruit	Granola and Fresh Fruit
LUNCH	Salad in a Jar	Salad in a Jar	Flatbread and Hummus with Veggies	Southwest Turbo Salad	Salad in a Jar
PM SNACK	Green Apple and Almond Butter	Green Apple and Almond Butter	Carrots and Almond Butter	Green Apple and Almond Butter	Carrots and Hummus
DINNER	Cobb Salad	Turkey Quinoa Bowl	Roasted Chicken Bites and Veggies	Baked Sweet Potato and Chicken Thighs	Pizza and Salad

✓	GROCERY LIST	QTY
☐	Packages of Strawberries (Freeze 1)	2
☐	Packages of Raspberries (Freeze 1)	2
☐	Package of Blackberries	1
☐	Package of Blueberries	1
☐	Oranges	4
☐	Lemon	1
☐	Lime	1
☐	Granny Smith Apples	4
☐	Bundle of Spotted Bananas	1
☐	Head of Leaf Lettuce	1
☐	Head of Romaine Lettuce	1
☐	Bunches of Spinach	2
☐	Celery Package	1
☐	Cucumbers	4
☐	Red Bell Peppers	5
☐	Green Bell Peppers	3
☐	Red Onions	3
☐	Yellow Onion	3
☐	Scallions	1

✓	GROCERY LIST	QTY
☐	Zucchinis	4
☐	Sweet Potatoes	2
☐	Carrots	4
☐	Baby Carrots	1
☐	Garlic Bulbs	2
☐	Tomato	1
☐	Cherry Tomatoes	1
☐	Avocados	3
☐	Fresh Cilantro	1
☐	Fresh Basil	1
☐	Fresh Parsley	5
☐	Organic Fermented Tofu	1
☐	Gallons of Coconut Milk	2.5
☐	Egg (Optional)	1
☑	Ground Flax	1
☐	Pine Nuts	1
☐	Almond Butter	1
☐	Chicken Breasts	3
☐	Chicken Thighs	4

✓	GROCERY LIST	QTY
☐	lb of Ground Turkey	1
☐	lb of Sliced Pepperoni	1
☐	Can of Black Beans	1

PANTRY STAPLES

Potato Starch	Red Chili Powder	Coriander
Coconut Flour	Red Pepper Flakes	Cacao
Quinoa	Turmeric	Aqua Fava (Bean Water)
Coconut Sugar	Diced Tomatoes	
Himalayn Salt	Diced Green Chilis	16oz of Chicken Broth
Pepper	Granola (Gluten Free)	

CONDIMENTS

Olive Oil	Apple Cider Vinegar	Spicy Mustard (Non-GMO/Sugar Free)
Grapeseed Oll	Balsamic Vinegar	
Coconut Oil	Hummus	
Tomato Sauce	Raw Honey	

GRANOLA

INGREDIENTS

- 2 Cups Quick Oats
- 3/4 Cup Chia or Flax Seeds
- 3/4 Cup Sunflower Seeds
- 1/2 Cup Almond Slivers
- 1/2 Cup Toasted Quinoa
- Hot Cereal
- 1 Tbsp Ginger, peeled and minced
- 1 Cup Dried Cranberries
- 1/3 Cup Coconut Sugar
- 1/3 Cup Maple Syrup
- 1/2 Cup Agave Nectar or

Honey
- 1/4 Cup Plant Based Butter
- 1 Tsp Ground Cinnamon
- 1/2 Tsp Ground Cardamom
- 1/4 Tsp Ground Cloves
- 1/2 Tsp Himalayan Salt
- 2 Tsp Vanilla Extract

DIRECTIONS

- Preheat oven to 400°.
- On a baking sheet with raised sides, stir together the oats, flax chia seeds, sunflower seeds, almonds and quinoa cereal. Bake 8 to 10 minutes, stirring often, until toasted.
- Remove from the oven, transfer to a large bowl and stir in the ginger and cranberries. Line a 11 x 13 inch baking dish with parchment paper and spray with non-stick spray.
- In a saucepan over medium heat, bring the coconut sugar, map syrup, and agave/ honey, butter, cinnamon, cardamom, cloves and salt to a simmer, stirring constantly. Remove from heat an

stir in the vanilla. Pour this mixture over the nut mixture and stir so everything is coated.

- Transfer to prepared baking dish and use a rubber spatula to spread out the mixture and press it into the pan. Place a sheet of wax or parchment paper on top and press down hard to compact the mixture into the pan. Let this cool in the pan for 2 to 3 hours, then turn out onto cutting board and use a large knife to cut into bars.

- Preheat oven to 300° and place the cut bars on a baking sheet lined with parchment paper. Bake for 20 minutes, or until the edges start to brown. Let cool completely, then store in an airtight container.

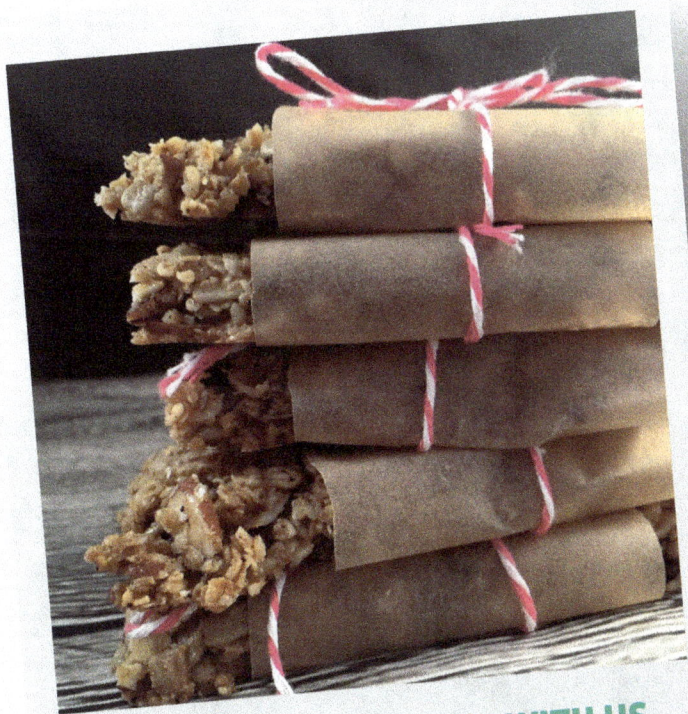

SHARE YOUR CREATIONS WITH US

#GFMOMCERTIFIED f P y in ▶ ⊙

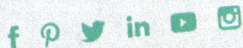

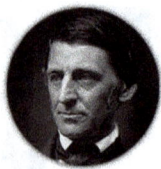

Ralph Waldo Emerson ✓
@ralphwaldoemerson

The first wealth is health.

FLATBREAD AND HUMMUS WITH VEGGIES

INGREDIENTS

- 1 Cup Potato Starch
- 1/4 Cup Coconut Flour
- 1/2 Cup Water
- 1/4 Cup Olive Oil
- 1 Tsp Garlic, Minced
- 1 Tsp Oregano
- 1/2 Tsp Coriander
- 1 Tsp Himalayan Salt
- 1/4 Cup Bean Water or 1 Egg
- 1 Red Pepper, thinly sliced
- 1 Green Pepper, thinly sliced
- 10 Baby Carrots

DIRECTIONS

- Preheat the oven to 450°. Line a cookie sheet or baking stone with parchment paper. Place the pan in the oven to get warm. In a large bowl, mix coconut flour, potato starch and pink salt. Stir in the warm water and olive oil and mix until combined. Let this set for 3-5 minutes. It will thicken up as the coconut flour absorbs the liquid. Add bean water (egg) and mix together with garlic, oregano and coriander.
- Remove the baking sheet from the oven and pour the flat bread dough on the parchment paper. Spread around.
- Cook for 20 minutes in the oven until the edges start to brown.
- Serve with veggies and hummus.

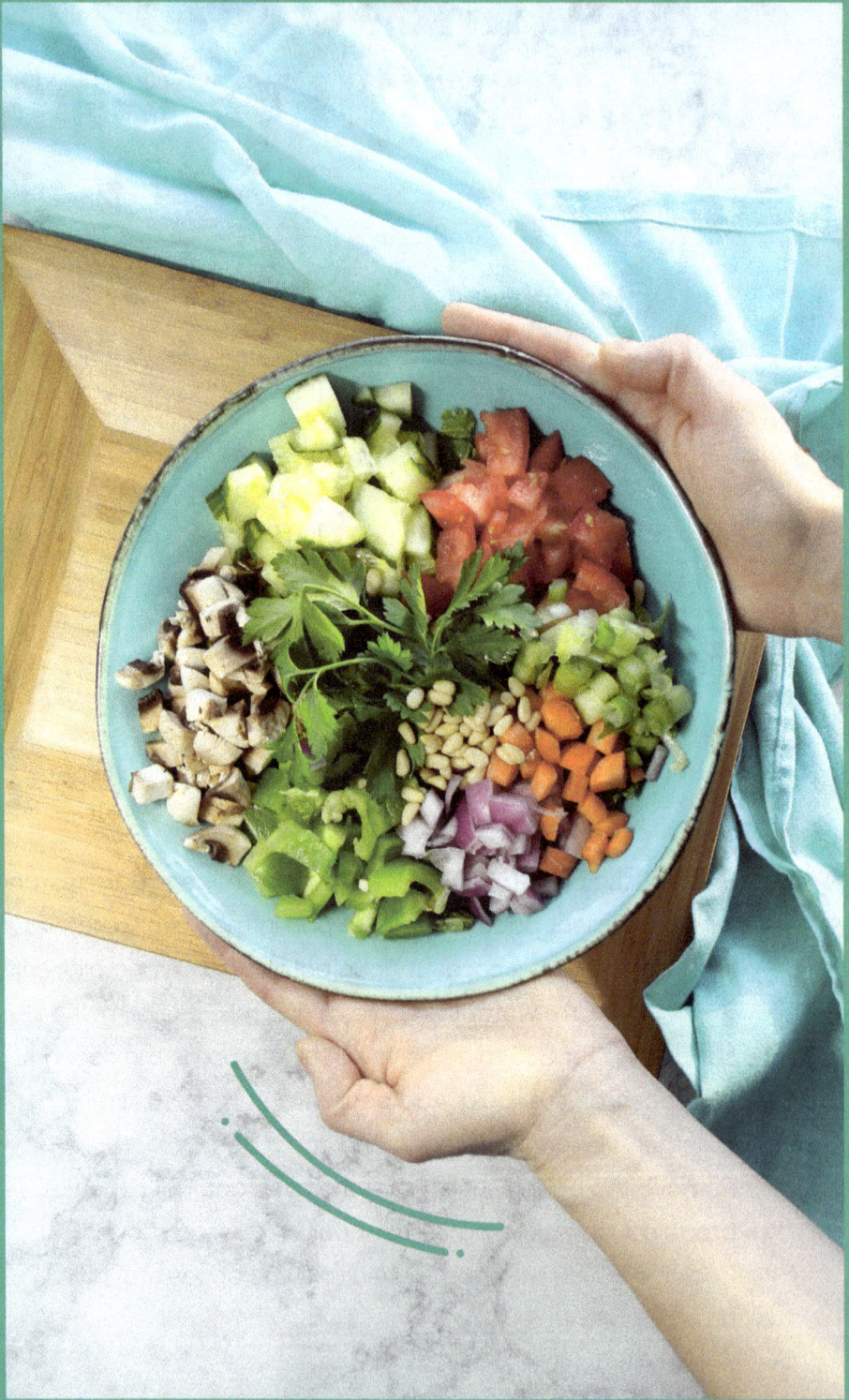

COBB SALAD

INGREDIENTS

- 1 4oz Chicken Breast, cut into 1" pieces Vegan - Replace with Mushrooms
- 1 Tbsp and 1 Tsp Extra Virgin Olive Oil
- 1 Tsp Apple Cider Vinegar
- 2 Tbsp Fresh Lemon
- 1 Garlic Clove, minced
- Dash of Himalayan Salt
- Dash of Black Pepper
- 1 Cucumber, peeled and diced
- 1 Green Pepper, diced
- 1 Tomato, diced
- 1/2 Red Onion, diced
- 1 Carrot, diced
- 1/4 Cup Fresh Parsley, torn
- 1 Scallion, thinly sliced
- 2 Cups Romain Hearts, Diced
- 1/4 Cup Pine Nuts

DIRECTIONS

- Toss chicken with 1 tsp oil, 1 Tbsp lemon juice, garlic, salt and pepper. In medium skillet cook chicken 7-8 minutes over medium-high heat or until cooked through. Place lettuce on a plate. Line up diced toppings in neat rows. Toss with 1 Tbsp lemon juice, 1 Tbsp oil, 1 tsp apple cider vinegar. Season with Himalayan salt and pepper to taste.

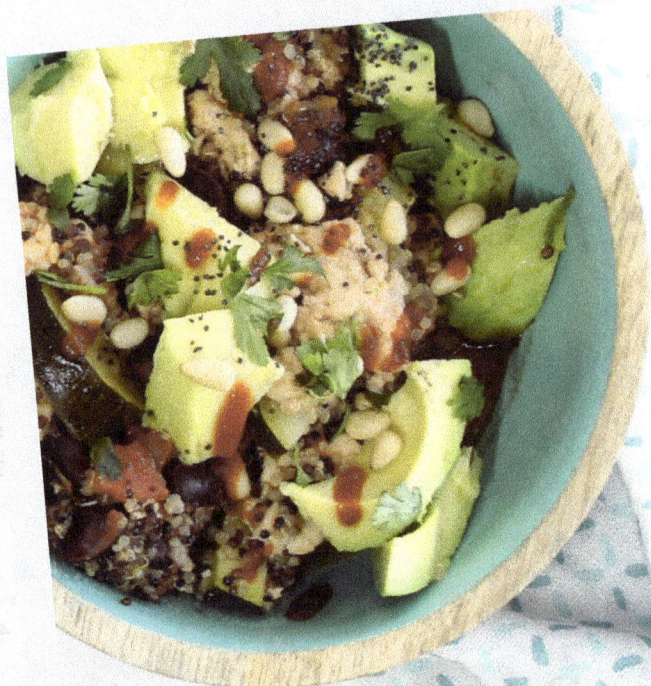

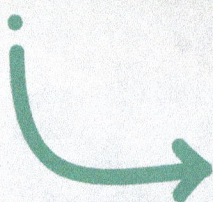

BON APPÉTIT!

TURKEY QUINOA BOWL

INGREDIENTS

- 1 Pound Ground Turkey
- 2 Tsp Extra Virgin Olive Oil
- 1 Yellow Onion, diced
- 2 Garlic Cloves, minced
- 1/2 Tsp Crushed Red Pepper Flakes
- 1 Tsp Herbal Seasoning
- 1 Tsp Himalayan Salt
- 1/2 Tsp Pepper
- 1 Can Diced Tomatoes, drained
- 1 Can Black Beans, drained and rinsed
- 2 Cups Zucchini, chopped
- 1 Cup Quinoa
- 2 Cups Chicken Broth
- 1 Can Diced Green Chiles
- 1/2 Cup Pine Nuts, toasted
- 1 Avocado, diced

DIRECTIONS

- In a large skillet heat oil over medium-high heat. Then add turkey, onion and garlic and saute until turkey is brown and onion is soft. Add red pepper flakes, herbal seasoning, salt and pepper; cook 1 minute. Stir in tomatoes, black beans, zucchini, pine nuts, quinoa and chicken broth; cover, reduce heat to medium-low and simmer for 15 minutes or until quinoa is cooked. Serve topped with avocado.

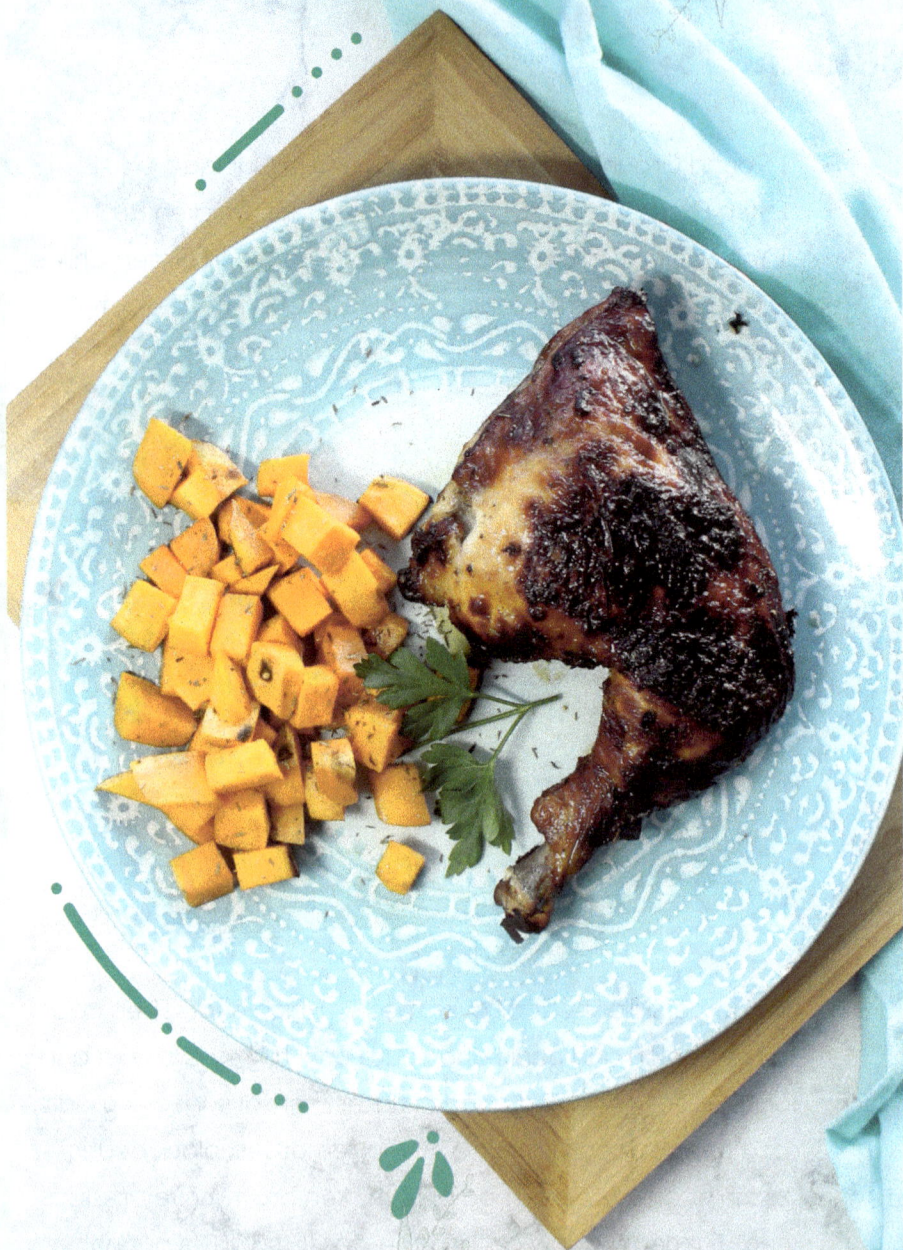

BAKED SWEET POTATO AND CHICKEN THIGHS

INGREDIENTS

- 2 Small Sweet Potatoes, pierced with a fork several times
- 4 Chicken Thighs, Bone In
- 2 Tsp Olive Oil
- 1 Tsp Ground Turmeric
- 1/2 Tsp Ground Coriander
- 1 Tsp Himalayan Salt

DIRECTIONS

- Preheat oven to 450°. Bake sweet potatoes for 40 minutes or until tender. Cut sweet potatoes almost in half lengthwise.
- Drizzle thighs with oil and sprinkle with spice mix. Bake on upper rack in oven with sweet potoatoes on baking sheet for 20 minutes, then flip back for 15 more minutes or until chicken is cooked completely.

JOURNAL EXERCISES

Q: What kind of food and activities will make my body shine?

Q: What do you most want to experience in your health?

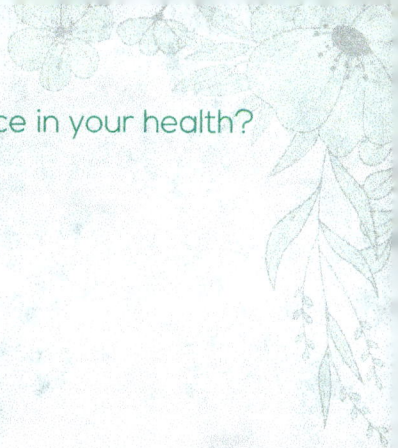

"BEGINNING IN ITSELF HAS NO VALUE, IT IS AN END WHICH MAKES BEGINNING MEANINGFUL, WE MUST END WHAT WE BEGUN."

– AMIT KALANTRI

BONUS WEEK

ADRENAL RESET

ADRENAL RESET MENU

	MON	TUE	WED	THU	FRI
BREAKFAST	Green Drink	Green Drink	Green Drink	Green Drink	Chocolate Banana Almond Smoothie
AM SNACK	Adrenal Berry Mix Salad	Adrenal Berry Mix Salad	Adrenal Berry Mix Salad	Adrenal Berry Mix Salad	Green Appl and Almon Butter
LUNCH	Salad in a Jar	Bok Choy Salad	Salad in a Jar	Salad in a Jar	Salad in a J
PM SNACK	Carrots and Almond Butter	Celery and Almond Butter	Green Apple and Almond Butter	Carrots and Almond Butter	Carrots an Almond Butter
DINNER	Lentil Minestrone Soup	Lentil Minestrone Soup	Roasted Fish and Sweet Potatoes	Veggie Stir-Fry	Pizza and Salad

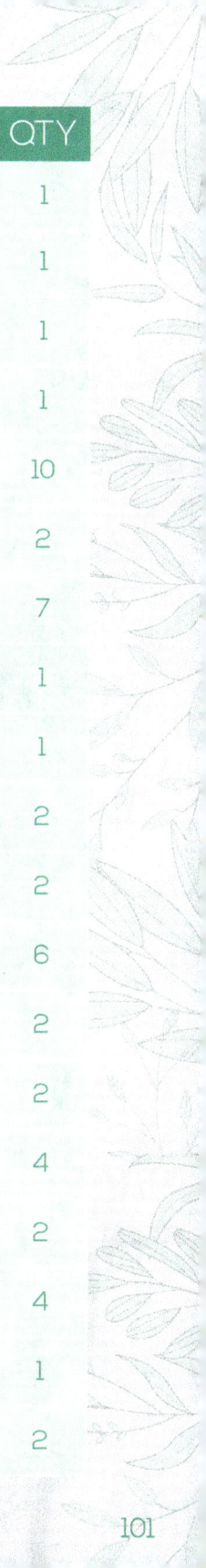

✓	GROCERY LIST	QTY
☐	Package of Strawberries	1
☐	Package of Raspberries	1
☐	Package of Blackberries	1
☐	Package of Blueberries	1
☐	Lemons	10
☐	Limes	2
☐	Granny Smith Apples	7
☐	Bundle of Spotted Bananas	1
☐	Grapes	1
☐	Pears	2
☐	Head of Leaf Lettuce	2
☐	Bok Choy	6
☐	Bunches of Spinach	2
☐	Packages of Celery	2
☐	Cucumbers	4
☐	Zucchinis	2
☐	Red Bell Peppers	4
☐	Green Bell Pepper	1
☐	Jalapeno Peppers (Optional)	2

✓	GROCERY LIST	QTY
☐	Red Onions	2
☐	Yellow Onion	1
☐	Scallions	1
☐	Sweet Potatoes	2
☐	Yellow Squash	2
☐	Carrots	10
☐	Baby Carrots	1
☐	Snap Peas	1
☐	Fresh Green Beans	1
☐	String Beans	1
☐	Fresh Ginger	1
☐	Broccoli Florets	1
☐	Radishes	1
☐	Garlic Bulbs	2
☐	Tomatoes	4
☐	Avocado	1
☐	Fresh Thyme	1
☐	Fresh Parsley	1
☐	Gallons of Coconut Milk	1.5

✓	GROCERY LIST	QTY
☐	Ground Flax	1
☐	Almond Butter	1
☐	Sliced Almonds	1

PANTRY STAPLES

Coconut Flour	Potato Starch	Chicken Bone Broth
Chili Powder	Green Tea	Red Pepper Flakes
Himalayn Salt	Cacao	Pepper
Oregano		

CONDIMENTS

Olive Oil	Apple Cider Vinegar	Spicy Mustard (Non-GMO/Sugar Free)
Grapeseed Oil	Balsamic Vinegar	
Coconut Oil	Rice Vinegar	
Raw Honey	Liquid Aminos	

GREEN DRINK

INGREDIENTS

- 3 Celery Stalks
- 1/2 Cucumber
- 1/2 Cup Parsley
- 1/2 Green Apple
- 1 Lemon with Skin

DIRECTIONS

- In a juicer - juice all ingredients OR

Peel lemon and rough chop all ingredients. Blend in high-speed blender with 1/2 cup water into juice.

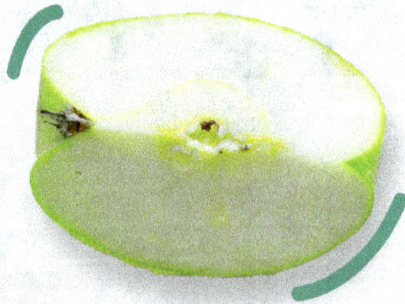

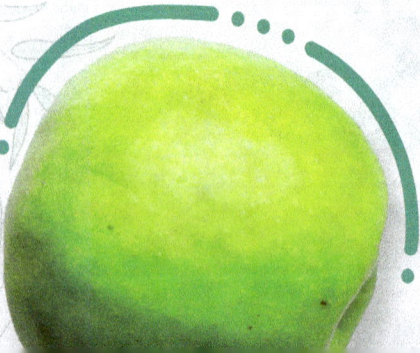

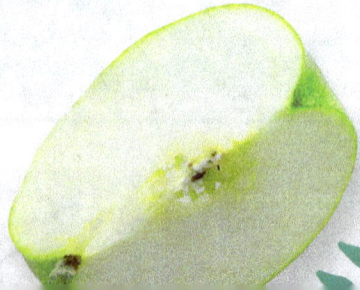

BOK CHOY SALAD

INGREDIENTS

- 6 Bok Choy, thinly sliced
- 1/2 Red Onion, sliced
- 1 Granny Smith Green Apple, diced
- 1 Lemon, juiced
- 1 Tsp Himalayan Salt
- 1/2 Tsp Coriander
- 1 Tbs Olive Oil

DIRECTIONS

- Combine all salad ingredients in large bowl. The veggies will get softer from the lemon juice/salt combo, so the longer you let it sit the better it tastes.
- Dress with olive oil before serving.

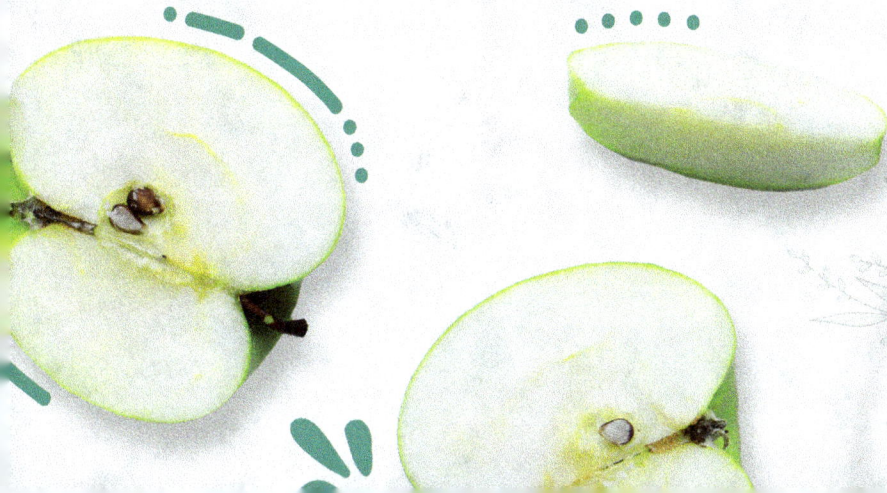

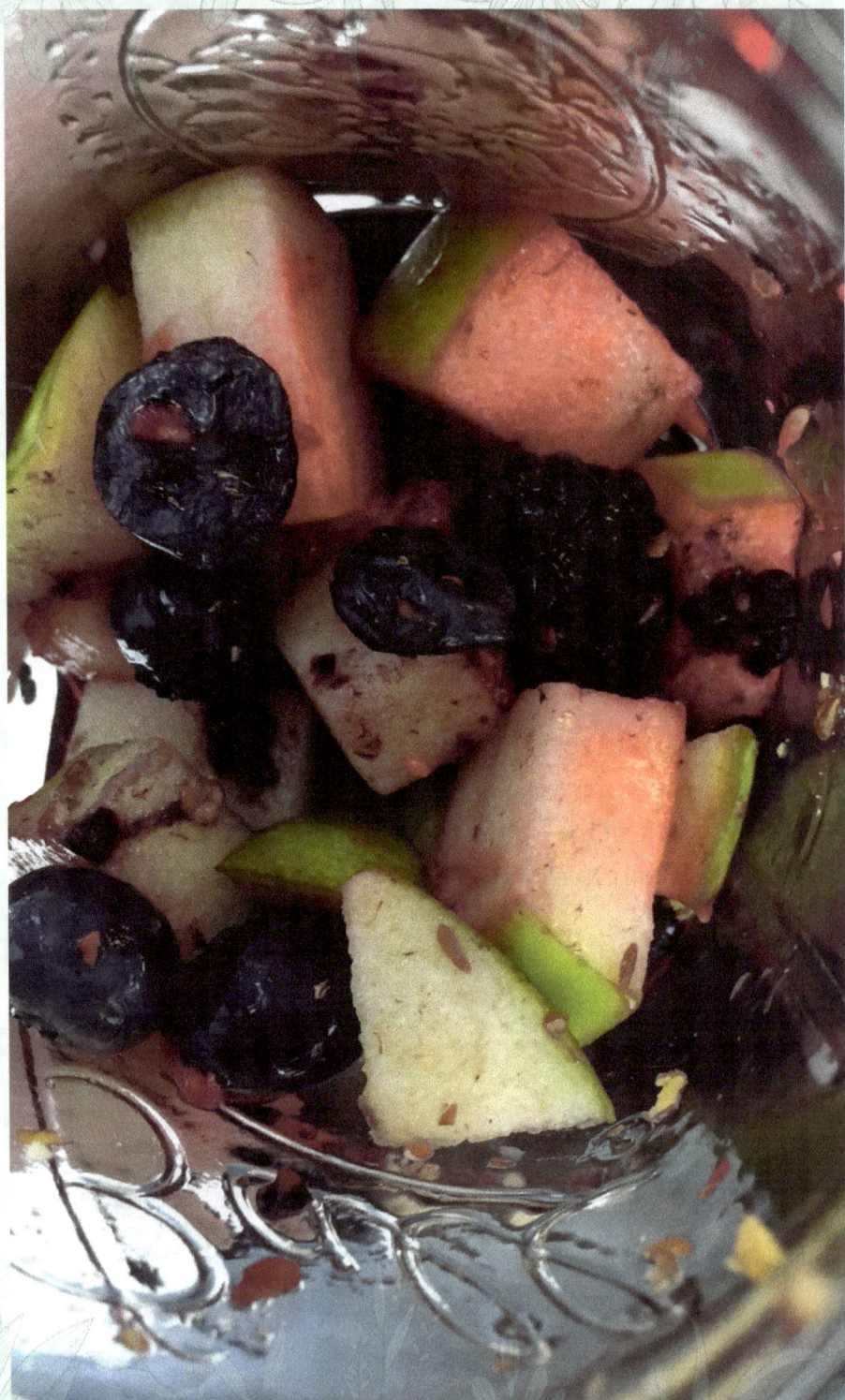

ADRENAL BERRY MIX SALAD

INGREDIENTS

- 1 Package Strawberries, rinsed and halved
- 1 Package Raspberries, rinsed
- 1 Package Blackberries, rinsed
- 1 Package Blueberries, rinsed
- 2 Green Apples, chopped
- 2 Pears, chopped
- 1 Cup Grapes
- 2 Tbsp Ground Flax

DIRECTIONS

- Mix all the berries and fruit together in a large bowl and store covered in the fridge.
- Single Serving
  - 1 Cup Salad
  - 1 Tsp Ground Flax
- *tip alert: Try and dry off as much water as possible. This will help the fruit last longer in the fridge.

LENTIL MINESTRONE SOUP

INGREDIENTS

- 1 Onion, chopped
- 2 Carrots, chopped
- 4 Cups Vegetable or Chicken Bone Broth
- 2 Zucchinis, chopped
- 2 Yellow Squashs, chopped
- 4 Tomatoes, chopped
- 1 Cup String Beans
- 1 Cup Lentils
- Himalayan Salt and Pepper to Taste
- Olive Oil

DIRECTIONS

- Boil a 2 quart pot of water, add lentils and cook for 15 minutes. Turn off and allow lentils to sit in water until soup is ready to add in.
- Saute 1 chopped onion in olive oil, salt and pepper for a few minutes in a large pot. Add a few chopped carrots and continue sauteing till fragrant. Then add 4 cups of vegetable or chicken bone broth and cook until carrots begin to soften. Add 2 chopped zucchinis and 2 chopped yellow squash, chopped tomatoes and string beans. Add lentils and cook on low till lentils are cooked.

ROASTED FISH

INGREDIENTS

- 4 White Fish Fillets
- 1 Small Bunch Fresh Thyme
- Juice of 2 Limes
- 4 Cloves Garlic, smashed
- 2 Jalapefio Peppers, halved, seeded and thinly sliced (optional)
- 1/2 Cup Grapeseed Oil
- 2 Tbsp Raw Honey
- 2 Tsp Himalayan Salt
- 1 Tsp Pepper

DIRECTIONS

- Strip thyme leaves from stems and combine with lime juice, garlic, jalapefio, oil, honey and salt in a large bowl. Add fish and turn to coat. Cover and marinate for 30 minutes at room temperature. Preheat oven to 400°. Put fish skin side up on a parchment lined rimmed baking sheet. Pour marinade on top, season with pepper. Roast the fish for 6 minutes. Rotate the pan 180°. Continue roasting the fish for 5 more minutes or until completely done.
- *tip alert: Halibut or Mahi Mahi are a great choice. For vegan feel free to substitute with tofu.

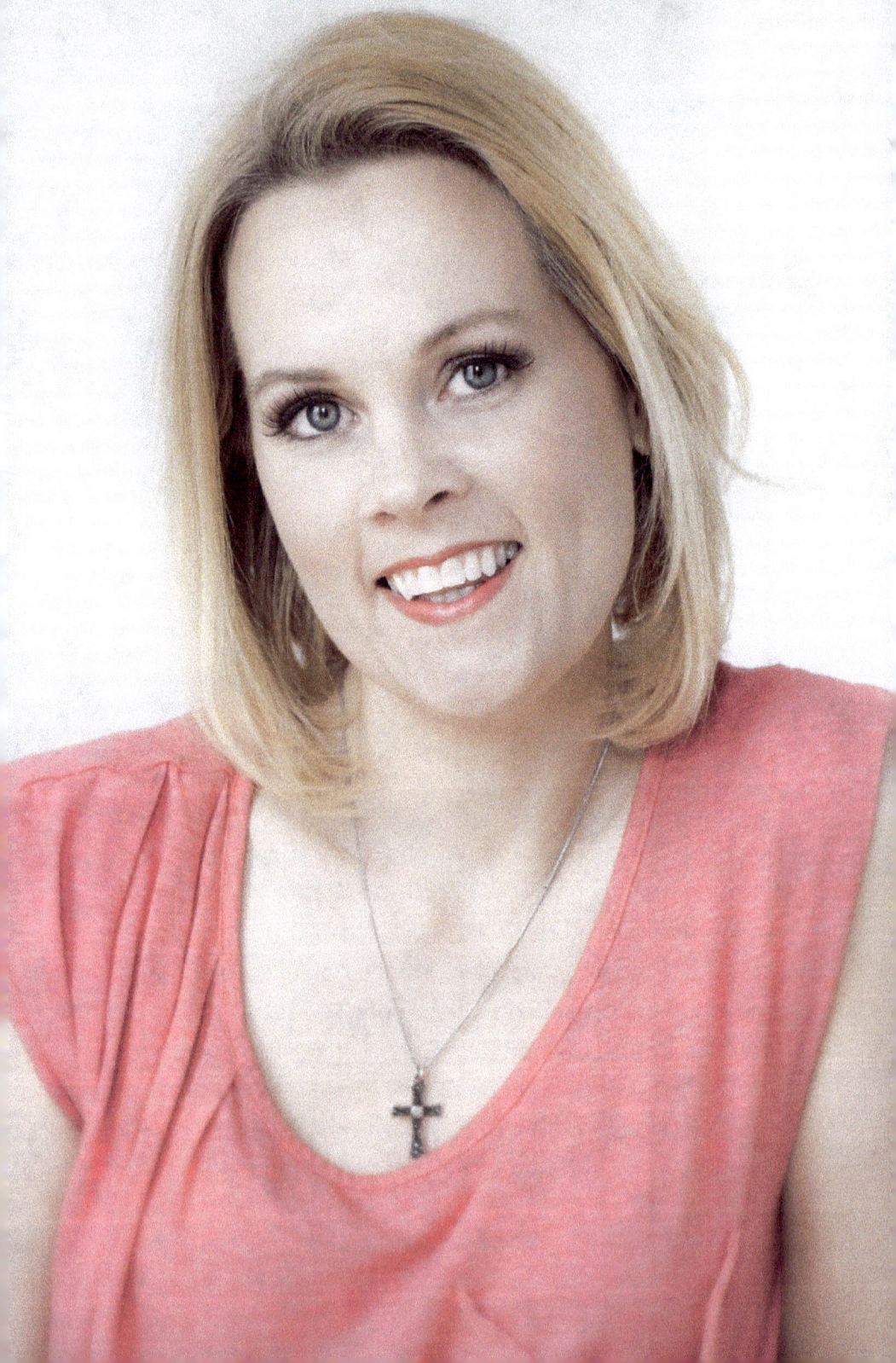

TIFFANY HINTON

Tiffany Hinton is the author of the #1 Amazon best-sellers Gluten Free Mom Certified and Mom Certified Celebrates Heritage and has written or contributed to over 16 allergen sensitive books. As a professional influencer, Hinton has developed upbeat, advocacy focused content for numerous brands such as Enjoy Life Foods, Lesser Evil, Just Thrive, Sunbutter and more and is a regular brand spokesman throughout the US including the award-winning Gluten Free and Allergen Friendly Expo, Nourished Festival, and Bloom Summit.

Tiffany has a compelling story that led to her gluten-free lifestyle. Tiffany is available for brand partnerships, speaking engagements, cooking demonstrations, content development, as well as healthy living promotional events.

She would be thrilled to work with any company that instills the same healthy lifestyle that she, America's favorite gluten-free Mom, promotes.

CONNECT WITH TIFFANY ON YOUR FAVORITE SOCIAL MEDIA PLATFORMS

GFMOMCERTIFIED.COM

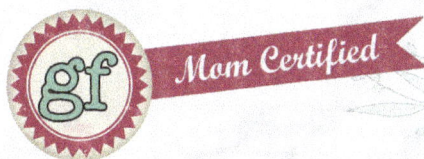

f P y in ▶ ◉

gf *Mom Certified*

NOTES

NOTES

NOTES

NOTES

NOTES

Editors: Tiffany Hinton and Anna Marie Imbordino
Graphic Design: Chicago Buzz Marketing
Photo Credits: Womanly Portraits, Life N Reflection
Photography, Chicago Buzz Marketing, and Tiffany Hinton

DISCLAIMER
This book is designed as a resource and inspirational recipe
book, made available to readers with the understanding that
the author and publisher are not offering any professional
medical advice specific to any individual's needs or
situations. The information provided is, in no way a substitute
for professional counsel, advice or treatment by a licensed
healthcare professional.

Because some ingredients and other products may interact
with certain health conditions or medications, or may
result in allergic or other reactions, always check with your
professional healthcare provider before incorporating new
foods into your diet. If you have any health conditions, you
are advised to have your health monitored regularly by
competent professionals who are familiar with your needs.
The author and publisher are not liable for any loss, injury
or damage that might arise from using the information
contained in this book or for any information that is not
included in its pages or scope.

Please note that products and companies mentioned in this
book are personal preferences of the author. Readers may
have different products and companies they prefer.

www.ingramcontent.com/pod-product-compliance
Lightning Source LLC
Chambersburg PA
CBHW071749270326
41928CB00013B/2849